Dr. Tooshi's High Fiber Diet

D1414823

Dr. Tooshi's High Fiber Diet

A Revolutionary Diet that will Help You to Lose Weight, Prevent Cancer, Heart Disease, Diabetes, and Digestive Disorders

Dr. A. Tooshi, Ph. D.

Writer's Showcase

San Jose New York Lincoln Shanghai

Dr. Tooshi's High Fiber Diet
A Revolutionary Diet that will Help You
to Lose Weight, Prevent Cancer, Heart
Disease, Diabetes, and Digestive Disorders

Writer's Showcase
an imprint of iUniverse.com, Inc.

For information address:
iUniverse.com, Inc.
5220 S 16th, Ste. 200
Lincoln, NE 68512
www.iuniverse.com

ISBN: 0-595-00191-2

Printed in the United States of America

Dedication

To my wife, Diane and my son, Michael for their encouragement.

Acknowledgments

Completion of this book would have been impossible without those individuals who participated in my diet program. I wish to acknowledge their motivation and commitment to improving their health and emotional well being. I am grateful to have had the opportunity to help thousands of overweight men and women who have shared their stories, frustrations and triumphs with me.

Sincere congratulations goes to Phyllis Joyce who lost 82 pounds and kept it off for more than ten years.

Special thanks are extended to Pat Lazar and Judy Woodward for their assistance in completion of this manuscript.

Preface

Many diet books have been written about losing weight. The major goals of these books have been how much and how fast to lose weight. However, no efforts have been made on how to maintain weight once a person has lost the desired amount and on educating the public in basic nutrition. Most Americans have very little knowledge in basic nutrition, and unfortunately, a lot of information regarding nutrition comes from newspaper reporters and tabloid magazine articles written by has-been movie stars or in-vogue celebrities, who have not taken even a basic nutrition course. Nutritional information from these sources can be very confusing and misleading. The problems of weight and obesity cannot be solved by diet pills, a crash diet or medications. The solution for such problems lies in a good, solid nutrition education. Education increases our horizon of thinking, reasoning and judgment. We can see the world in a wider range and we become more aware of ourselves and our environment. We recognize that our environment is changing rapidly and it is effecting our lives—the way we work, eat, exercise and the way we respond to stress in life. Such changes have caused a significant deterioration in our health and well-being. Today there is a tremendous rise in cardiovascular diseases, cancer, obesity, digestive disorders and many other health risks. We are trying desperately to find a magic drug to take care of these problems. However, we have failed badly in this war. We failed to understand that the problems of weight and obesity are the problems of a modern world. Chemical additives, high fat, and high salt, high sugar intake and lack of exercise are the major contributing factors to these problems. To succeed we must change our lifestyle; the way we eat and the way we work.

After twenty-five years of teaching nutrition on both graduate and undergraduate levels and managing a successful diet clinic for eighteen years, I have decided to write this book to provide people with a good understanding of nutrition as well as a proper diet plan. It is my hope that this plan will help those who need to lose weight and maintain it for many years to come. An effective diet plan and the necessary instructions that have helped thousands of my overweight patients through the years has been organized in a simple way in these pages. Once you have achieved your ideal weight, you are not left alone to fight a weight gain. I have organized an excellent, nutritional education program in this book as well as an effective maintenance program, which will help you for the rest of your healthier and productive life.

By the time you finish reading this book your nutritional knowledge will be more than your doctors. You will be able to select food items more wisely and plan your own diet in such a way that not only will you prevent weight gain, but you may prevent many chronic diseases as well. In this book I have provided a solid nutrition education, including the five divisions of nutrition, namely carbohydrates, proteins, fats, vitamins, minerals and water. Their functions, sources, requirements and deficiencies are discussed in detail.

In addition, a major section of this book has been devoted to:

1. A diet plan to lose weight and keep it off.
2. More food selections to choose from so that you do not get bored and become prone to nutritional deficiency.
3. Demonstrating that there is no need to measure or weigh food.
4. Easy and quick meal preparation.
5. Special information has been provided for eating out.
6. Individual weight loss, whether you need to lose 5 pounds, 10 pounds, 20 pounds or more. For each group, a special diet has been planned.

7. Well organized maintenance diets for after you achieve your goal, so that you can keep excess weight off for many years to come.

8. A special one day diet to help if you gain 2 or 3 pounds after attending a party or wedding. This one day diet will get rid of those 2 or 3 pounds within one day.

9. Some very healthy and delicious recipes.

Contents

Chapter 1

Chapter 2

Chapter 3

Chapter 4

Chapter 5

Chapter 6

Chapter 7

Chapter 8

Chapter 9

Chapter 10

Chapter 11

Chapter 12

Chapter 13

Chapter 14

Chapter 15

CHAPTER 1

INTRODUCTION

We may live in a modern world with television, radio, cars and airplanes, wear the latest fashion clothing and have the best medical science; but, the body we have is that of primitive man and woman. We may have traveled a long road from the cave dwellers in many ways through technology and education but the way our body handles factors such as air pollution, disease and food has changed very little. We have the body and brain of our ancestors who lived 150,000 years ago. Although our bodies and brains have remained virtually the same, the world around us has greatly changed, especially in the last hundred years. The Industrial Revolution has brought about a great advantage to the people in developed countries.

In contemporary society we have an abundant supply of food, massive transportation systems, communication networks to distribute data, household conveniences, high speed cooking, dish washing, air conditioning, the best heating system and many other amenities. But with these advantages have come water pollution, smog, food additives, chemical contamination of food supplies, as well as a lack of physical activities. Our cave-dweller bodies are not prepared to deal with these problems. We received, from our mothers and fathers, the genes that determine how our body works and responds to the world surrounding us. Many of these genes are thousands of years old and have not changed since our ancestors walked this earth. It is important that you understand the capacity of your body to deal with these changes.

Food was not always available to cavemen. They had to walk miles, sometimes over mountains, through valleys or climb trees to find food and water. In today's world we do not climb trees nor do we walk miles to obtain food. We have a tremendous supply of food and we make very little effort to obtain it.

Health as defined by the World Health Organization is the state of complete physical, mental and social well-being, not merely the absence of disease. Nutrition is the science of foods. It involves the actions, interactions and balance in relationship to health and disease. It is the processes by which the body ingests, digests, absorbs, transports, utilizes nutrients and disposes of the end products. Nutrients are the constituents in the food that must be supplied to the body in suitable amounts. These include protein, carbohydrates, fatty acid, minerals, vitamins and water. Knowledge of nutrition and its application in helping people select and obtain food for the primary purpose of nourishing their body, shows us that food has played a vital role in the rise or the decline of nations because of its effect on health and efficiency throughout history. Since earliest times food has been considered very important in the light of cause and cure of disease. The ancient Egyptians medical writings dating back to 1500 B.C. contain numerous recommendations for the cure, through food, of all kinds of ailments from headaches to baldness, diabetes and blindness.

Of all the factors which influence our lives and upon which our health and illness depend, undoubtedly the nature of our food is the most important one. We have all experienced how the strength of our muscles, our vigor, and our whole emotional tone and thinking is affected by the nature of what we eat. The food we eat must contain the essential nutrients in the right proportion. Our food must be mixed, varied and alternating. Our diet becomes nutritionally balanced when there is a due proportion of substances belonging to carbohydrate, protein and fat. History shows us that when food is insufficient and not diversified, the capacity of people to work is low and their body strength and mental health declines. There is no difference between a deficiency in diet and malnutrition. Few people realize that malnutrition is a pathological state. It is caused by (A) a relative, absolute deficiency or excess of one or more essential nutrients, (B) overeating , and (C) imbalanced diet which results from the lack of specific nutrients such as vitamins and minerals.

In view of the great advances in the science of nutrition, it is paradoxical that so much malnutrition exists in America today. It must be realized that almost all chronic diseases such as heart disease, diabetes, cancer and digestive disorders, especially obesity are rooted in what we eat. Food represents the crossroads of tradition, religion, habits and emotion. Recent changes in the social atmosphere within the United States have had an influential impact on national food habits. It is conceivable that the process of Americanization, specifically that involving the intermarriage of many nationalities, has resulted in considerable interchange of dietary customs, ideas and habits.

One social change that has the most far reaching effect has been the shift of American culture from agricultural life to industrial and urban existence. This single event has not only resulted in a considerable shift from the production of food at home, but has also influenced the decline of eating at home to the use of fast foods, restaurants and cafes. Lunch counters have become part of American life. One of the most common effects on changes in food habits is the tremendous size in the number of overweight population.

There has been a decrease in the total consumption of carbohydrates within the past 65 years. In 1912, people consumed approximately 500 grams of carbohydrates per day. Now, this consumption has dropped to approximately 360 grams per day in 1990. This decrease in carbohydrate consumption is mainly due to less intake of complex carbohydrate which are rich sources of fiber and has resulted in the lack of fiber in the American diet. No longer can we ignore the importance of fiber in the health and well-being of every individual. The disappearance of fiber from our diet is being scrutinized as a major contributing factor in the etiology of common non-infectious diseases such as colon cancer, diabetes, diverticulitis, heart disease and constipation.

OBESITY

Every cell in the body is like a living organism. Each cell's basic requirements consist of oxygen, nutrients, and water and the removal of metabolic waste. The cells acquire these materials, combine them together, and produce energy and building materials for the entire body. This process is carried out by the cardiovascular and respiratory systems. Therefore we need a strong heart, a healthy network of blood vessels, and efficient lungs to push the blood through hundreds of obstacles to reach every cell. One of the major obstacles to blood circulation is body fat. Body fat slows down circulation and reduces the speed of delivery of needed materials to vital organs such as the brain, kidneys, liver and the heart muscle itself.

Obesity is increasing at an alarming extent in America. Some thirty-five percent of all teenagers and fifty-five percent of all adults are overweight.

Obesity can be divided into two categories:
1. Childhood Obesity
2. Adulthood Obesity

Children who become overweight will grow and develop adequate muscles and bones, but they will have more body fat than normal children. These overweight children are less likely to be able to reduce weight as successfully as people who become overweight at adulthood. Early onset obesity is believed to be resistant to dietary treatment because fat cell development mainly takes place during the period of infancy up to two years of age and again during the pre-adolescence stage of nine to ten years of age. These are very critical periods of a child's life. If a child consumes more food during these periods then more fat cells will develop. Such a child will have a serious problem to lose weight in the future.

Today, the relation between obesity and disease has been clearly demonstrated. The incidence of heart disease, cancer, diabetes and lung disease is forty percent higher among overweight people than within the normal weight population. Life expectancy and age specific death rates are increased ten percent for each ten pounds of excess weight. Therefore an excess of twenty-five pounds will reduce life expectancy by twenty-five percent. In the final analysis, obesity results from overeating in relation to one's physiological and environmental requirements. In animal studies, caloric restriction has improved survival rate and reduced the risk of cancer in mice and has prolonged greatly the life expectancy of animals. Caloric restriction has also reduced the incidence of diabetes and hypertension in humans. The principle causes of death among obese individuals are cardiovascular and renal disorders, diabetes, liver, and gall bladder diseases. A gain in body weight is often accompanied by changes in serum lipids, blood pressure, uric acid and carbohydrate tolerance. However, a reduction in body weight often results in a reduction of serum cholesterol, diabetes, cancer and blood pressure. According to scientific studies almost ninety percent of all human diseases are rooted in poor nutrition. Heart disease, high blood pressure, high cholesterol, diabetes, cancer, and digestive diseases such as stomach gas, bloatedness, constipation, acid reflux, and gall bladder can be prevented by increasing the consumption of high fiber foods. Fiber is the indigestible part of carbohydrates. Humans are not capable to digest fiber due to lack of a specific enzyme called amylase and therefore it must be excreted through the feces. However, animals such as cows and horses can break down and utilize fiber as a source of energy.

Fiber can only be obtained from plants. Good sources of fiber are fruits, vegetables, rice, potatoes, legumes, and grain products. The beneficial effect of eating a high fiber diet is mainly to reduce the body weight and to promote health.

The problem with the poor eating habits of Americans is rooted in our inability to take action. Today there is a gap between knowledge and action. This gap is continuously increasing as our knowledge in nutrition increases. Today, we have far more information concerning the connection between high fat foods and heart disease, cancer and weight gain. Despite this knowledge, people still continue to eat high fat foods. Questions about preventive medicine do not concern a lack of knowledge. We do not take action or responsibility to improve our health.

Many of our food habits are based in our cultural and childhood habits, not on conscious decision making. We learned these food habits from our parents at an early age and they have become increasingly woven into the fabric of our current eating habits. In order to become aware of the harmful effects our habits have on our health, it requires a conscious effort to examine our food habits from the perspective of our health and to make a serious effort to change them. The human body and mind are extremely flexible. Poor health habits can be overcome by our enormous adaptability. It is only too easy to decide to change one's lifestyle tomorrow or the next day, but not now. Too often people do not value health until they lose it. With the pressure of day to day living, it is difficult to take time out to examine our habits from this perspective, but it is an important step in assuming responsibility for our well-being.

CAUSES OF OBESITY

Obesity is caused by genetic and environmental factors. Environmental factors such as stress, loneliness, boredom, depression and social gathering, all play a vital role in the over-consumption of food. Food consumption that causes obesity is also related to three factors:

1. Quantity of the food (how much you eat at one time).
2. Frequency of eating (how often you consume food).
3. Quality of food (the types of food you eat is very important). Do you consume high fat foods or low fat foods that are rich in fiber? It is important to know that the size of a meal plays an important role in weight gain. A large meal contributes to weight gain, whereas a small meal helps to bring about a weight loss.

In America, the majority of overweight people are the products of environmental influences, not genetic. Individuals eat more and exercise less. Most of these people had a normal childhood, their weight was normal, their level of exercise was excellent, and their eating habits were good. By the time they arrived at the age of twenty, they had a normal body weight. After the age of twenty, the growth process ceases and the aging process begins. At this stage of life, three major forces affect our body:

1. Metabolism declines. The cell's capacity to consume more energy is reduced.
2. Our level of activity declines as people accept the responsibility of work and family.
3. Social activity and contact increases, contributing to more eating.

As a result of these three major forces we are continually exposed to a weight gaining process and our population is becoming obese. It is important to be aware that there are very few genetically overweight people in America. If you look back to the years spanning 1920 to 1930, we find most people in America, men, women and children, were underweight. There were not as many obese people as you find today because food was not as plentiful and daily life was full of physical activity. They had very few cars, fewer home appliances and very little time for leisure activities. Life for them was very active.

DANGER OF OBESITY

Obesity places a tremendous physical limitation on people. Limitations may include difficulty in walking, climbing stairs, getting into and out of automobiles, and various other physical activities. In warm weather, people who are overweight become more uncomfortable because their added body fat creates insulation making it difficult to control heat and temperature in the body. A lack of temperature control puts a tremendous load on the heart and lungs making it very hard to circulate the blood. Excessive body weight increases the effort of breathing because of the additional work in moving the thoracic cage, abdomen and diaphragm. Therefore, an overweight person breathes less air into the lungs and in turn exhales less air. Less efficient breathing increases carbon dioxide in the blood and causes circulatory problems as well as physical and mental fatigue. People with excessive weight are also prone to chronic illnesses such as high blood pressure, renal disease, diabetes, gout, gall bladder, heart disease and cancer. The life expectancy of people who are overweight is much shorter than people of normal weight. It is well stated that "the longer the belt line, the shorter the life line". Data from insurance companies also supports this notion. If a person is ten percent above the average normal weight, the chances to die early is more than twenty percent. The mortality rate for specific diseases such as heart disease is twenty percent above average and for stroke, it is fifty percent above average. When the overweight factor combines with one or more other diseases such as high blood pressure, high cholesterol, diabetes or heart disease the effect on mortality is even higher.

WHAT IS ADIPOSE TISSUE

Adipose tissue is made up from fat cells and is composed of about 72 percent fat, 23 percent water, and a very small amount of other chemicals. The number of fat cells that exist in the body has been determined by the time a person reaches the age of nine or ten; and they remain fixed throughout life. Fat cells can increase in size leading to obesity. Weight reduction programs can only reduce the size of the cells, but not the number of the cells.

There are two major characteristics of adipose tissue:

1. It slows down the speed of blood flow, resulting in the reduction of the delivery of nutrients to the other tissues.
2. It holds a large amount of blood volume, thus reducing the amount of blood available to nourish the other tissues.

Both characteristics of adipose tissue not only reduce the metabolism of the body, but also reduce the energy production of the body. Consequently, the body weight will be increased. We must be aware that obesity usually begins when there is a drastic change in lifestyle such as the change from home to college life, from college to the job market, from single life to married life and after pregnancy. All these are periods in life when weight gain commonly takes place. Knowing that weight gain may occur allows a person to become more conscious of the potential to gain weight and to monitor one's eating and exercise habits. When a person does not pay attention to these changes, he or she will gain weight. When people gain weight they want to lose it as soon as possible and as fast as they can. It does not always matter to them what kind of diet, pills, medications, foods, good or poor diet, safe or unsafe method they choose; they just do not care.

We must change our lifestyle if we are going to be successful in this battle. However, our lifestyle must be changed gradually. That means we need to consume less calories, increase physical activity and control factors influencing eating. The problem remains that most overweight people prefer not to change their lifestyle. They look for an easy way of losing weight and there are many diets from which to choose, each promising a drastic weight loss. Some of these diets are extremely harmful for those people who resist change. They become easy prey to the empty promises of these junk diets. The major problem of weight loss is how to keep it off after you lose the weight.

A successful weight loss program must have the following characteristics:
1. It allows you significant weight loss while providing a well balanced diet, containing essential nutrients, vitamins and minerals.
2. It provides you with a good maintenance diet, allowing you to follow it for many years into the future.

There is no miracle diet, no quick scheme, no easy way out. We must control our calorie consumption according to the laws of thermodynamics, which states that "calories cannot be created and calories cannot be destroyed". This means that a calorie can only change its form. For example, the calories in an apple are chemical calories stored in the apple. When we eat the apple, the calories enter our body. These calories must be utilized, otherwise unused calories will store in the body causing weight gain.

There are three ways the body uses calories:
1. Mechanical activities such as physical activities.
2. Thermal activities to produce heat in the body.
3. Electrical activities such as sending nerve impulses to the various parts of the body.

Two ways we can control our weight:
1. By increasing the level of physical activity.
2. By consuming fewer calories.

CARDIOVASCULAR SYSTEM AND OBESITY

The cardiovascular system is made up from the heart and the blood vessels, which are termed arteries, veins and capillaries.

The Heart

The heart is a hollow muscular organ lying slightly to the left of the mid line of the chest. It works as a pump, supplying blood to every cell and organ in the body. It beats twenty-four hours a day without any rest or stop. The heart is a very strong muscle, having a tremendous forcing ability to push the blood through thousands of miles of blood vessels.

The heart has two actions:

1. Contraction: This action enables the heart to force blood out of the heart chambers to the blood vessels.
2. Relaxation: This action allows blood to get inside the heart. The combination of contraction and relaxation of the heart is called a pulse or a heart rate.

On average, the heart of a man beats 72 times per minute and a woman's heart beats 76 times per minute. The heartbeat is sensitive to the following factors:

1. Stress. Stress increases the resting pulse rate.
2. Lack of exercise. Sedentary people have a higher pulse rate than those who are physically active.
3. Body weight. Excessive body weight increases the resting pulse rate.
4. Meditation and relaxation. It reduces the resting pulse rate.

The Body Weight

When a person gains weight, body fat increases, fat penetrates inside the heart muscle, and it gradually weakens the strength and forcing ability of the heart. When such a condition occurs, the heart no longer provides an adequate amount of blood to the tissues.

As a result:

1. Metabolism goes down.
2. Resting pulse rate goes up.

3. Blood pressure goes up.

4. Energy production is impaired.

5. Ability of a person to work and exercise deteriorates.

The Blood Vessels and The Body Weight:

Arteries circulate blood throughout the body. They nourish every cell and tissue with oxygen and nutrients. They remove waste products away from the body. Arteries have certain characteristics that make them able to carry on the circulation of the blood. The arteries consist of a smooth inner lining covered largely by elastic fibers, which absorb the pulsation of the heart. As the heart beats, the elastic arterial walls make the strong pulsation into a nearly constant blood pressure. Blood passes through the arteries at the speed of 15.6 inches per second when the body is at rest. During exercise the speed of blood circulation goes up. When the blood pressure goes up, the arteries expand like rubber to accommodate a larger amount of blood flowing without any problem. When a person gains weight, fat and cholesterol accumulate in the walls of the arteries. The arteries lose elasticity and no longer expand. They become hardened. When blood pressure goes up, the force of the blood pressure breaks the hardened arteries causing stroke or heart attack.

BLOOD PRESSURE AND BODY WEIGHT

Blood pressure is the pressure of the blood against the walls of the blood vessels. This pressure is generated by the heart during its contraction. Blood pressure is determined by several interrelated factors including:

1. The pumping action of the heart.

2. Resistance to the blood flow by the arteries.

3. The elasticity of the walls of the arteries.

4. Blood volume.

5. The blood viscosity or blood thickness.

During each heartbeat, the artery expands and absorbs the increase in blood pressure. When the heart relaxes in preparation for another beat, the aortic valve closes to prevent blood from flowing back to the heart chambers and the artery walls spring back, forcing the blood through the body between contractions. In this way the arteries act as a chamber on the pulsation and provide a steady flow of blood through the blood vessels. Because of this, there are two blood pressures within the blood vessels during one complete heartbeat. A high blood pressure during the contraction of the heart and a lower blood pressure during the relaxation of the heart occurs. These two blood pressures are called systolic and diastolic blood pressures respectively.

Factors Affecting Blood Pressure:

1. Exercise. During physical activity, blood pressure goes up. It comes back to the resting state when exercise stops.

2. Stress. Mental stress elevates both systolic and diastolic blood pressures.

3. Body Weight. An increase in body weight increases blood pressure. After weight loss, blood pressure drops.

4. Salt. A high consumption of salt increases water retention in the body causing increased blood pressure.

Fiber has several protective qualities. Its effect in stool bulk, softness and transit time is believed to play a major role in:

1. Lowering the blood pressure.

2. Reducing the exposure of the gut's mucous to carcinogenic substances in the feces

3. Lessening colon pressure that may lead to diverticulitis.

Fiber binds with bile acids leading to an increased cholesterol degradation and excretion through the feces. Reduction in the levels of blood cholesterol also prevents hardening of the arteries, high blood pressure and heart disease.

What Is A Normal Blood Pressure?

A systolic blood pressure of 120 and a diastolic blood pressure of 80 are normal.

Low Blood Pressure:

A systolic blood pressure of 90 and a diastolic blood pressure below 60 are considered to be low blood pressure. Low blood pressure is an indication of:

1. Poor circulation.
2. A weak heart, not capable of producing a strong force to push the blood through the blood vessels.
3. People with low blood pressure have no energy. They feel tired most of the time. They have very little endurance during exercise.

High Blood Pressure:

Systolic blood pressure over 130 and diastolic blood pressure over 90 are considered a high blood pressure. High blood pressure is caused by:

A) A weak heart. A heart that can not produce a strong force during contraction.
B) Poor blood vessels. Blood vessels that are hardened by cholesterol and have lost their elasticity. They can no longer expand during high blood pressure.
C) Water retention. Retaining fluid puts pressure on the arteries, creating resistance to blood flow. As a result of that pressure, the blood pressure goes up.
D) Excessive body weight. There is a correlation between body weight and high blood pressure. You can lower blood pressure by losing weight.

Blood Pressure And Weight

When a person gains weight, two major problems confront the cardiovascular system.

1. Excessive body weight puts extra pressure on the arteries, reducing the flow of blood.

2. Weight gain accompanies a large amount of water retention. The accumulation of this water in the body also reduces the flow of blood in the tissues.

From the above discussion, it is clear that body weight and water retention are responsible for high blood pressure.

METABOLISM

Metabolism encompasses all the chemical changes that occur in living organisms in the course of their vital activities. These changes are:

1. Catabolism
2. Anabolism

Catabolism refers to processes by which nutrients and cellular substances are broken down into simple compounds resulting in the liberation of energy. Anabolism is the process in which new tissues and cells are built by energy that has been liberated through the catabolic process. The leftover energy is stored as fat.

WHAT IS ENERGY

Energy is defined as the power to do work. Energy exists in many forms, all of which are inter-convertible. For example, the energy of an apple is a chemical energy, but when it is digested in the human body, the apple's energy can be converted into:

1. Mechanical Energy to perform physical work.
2. Chemical Energy to perform chemical activities.
3. Heat Energy to maintain the body temperature.
4. Electrical Energy to send nerve impulses.
5. Stored Energy (fat) in the body.

The availability of energy and the amount of it has become a very important issue in our times. Whether it be the oil, gas, coal or electrical energy to heat our homes, drive our cars or run our factories; or whether in direct human terms, it is the amount of available foods to provide energy to accomplish the chemical, biological and physical activities of our body. Sufficient food to meet the energy requirements of our body is the first nutritional priority. When the supply of energy is low, the capacity to work deteriorates and, in children, growth is retarded or ceased. All energy comes from plants and animal foods we eat. Carbohydrates, fats and proteins are the energy yielding substances. The energy value of foods and energy exchanges of the body are expressed in terms of the calorie. By definition, a calorie is the amount of heat required to raise the temperature of one kilogram (kg.) of water one degree centigrade (c).

Basal Metabolism

Basal metabolism is the amount of energy required to carry on the activities of the body in the resting state. It includes the functional activities of the various organs such as the brain, heart, liver, kidneys, lungs, digestive system and glands as well as other activities including oxidation of foods and maintenance of the body temperature.

Factors Influencing The Basal Metabolism

1. Age—The basal metabolism is at the highest rate during the first two years of life. It declines gradually throughout childhood and then rises in adolescence. Thereafter the decline continues throughout life.
2. Sleep—During the sleep hours, the basal metabolism is about ten percent lower than in the waking state.
3. Digestion—During the digestion of food, metabolism goes up. The activities of the digestive system, including the digestion and elimination processes, increase the metabolism of the body. Food such as protein and fat take a longer time to be digested whereas carbohydrate foods take less time.

4. Pregnancy—During the last trimester of pregnancy the total metabolism increases by fifteen to twenty-five percent. This increase is due to the increase in weight of women and the high rate of metabolism of the fetus.

5. Muscular Activity—Physical activity increases the basal metabolism because activity increases lean body mass and reduces the fat content of the body. Muscle tissues (lean body mass) utilize more energy than fatty tissues. An athlete with less body fat will have a higher basal metabolic rate than an overweight person.

6. Glands—Endocrine glands such as the thyroid gland regulate the rate of energy metabolism. Any changes in thyroid activity is reflected in the metabolic rate. If the thyroid is overactive, the metabolism may speed up as much as 75 to 100 percent. If the activity of the gland is decreased, the metabolism is decreased by 30 to 40 percent.

7. Body Fat—The metabolism of fatty tissues is very low, especially when a person gains weight the basal metabolism goes down. As a result of weight gain, the body cannot utilize the food energy properly and the person will keep gaining weight until the energy intake is reduced.

BODY COMPOSITION AND BODY TYPES

Obesity can be defined as weighing at least twenty percent more than the desired body weight, whereas overweight is defined as ten percent over the desired body weight. Scientific studies show that genetics play a very important role in the body types regarding:

1. Body Shape
2. Amount of Fatty Tissue
3. Distribution of fat in the body

Each person inherits his or her body type and shape.

There are three major body types:
1. Ectomorphy
2. Mesomorphy
3. Endomorphy

Ectomorphy

This group has a very easy time to control their body weight. They have a high basal metabolism and burn food calories much faster than the other body types. They stay relatively thin throughout life. They live longer and they are genetically active. Their immune system is very strong and they can fight infection and disease better than others. There are some extreme ectomorphics. They are very thin, always feel tired, have stress and sleeping disorders. Many of them have digestive disorders. They have a problem of absorbing foods. This group requires considerable health counseling with respect to an adequate diet, exercise, body building activities, relaxation, meditation and a stress management program.

Endomorphy

Endomorphics are an extremely ponderous, soft-fleshed type. Primary characteristics include rounded shoulders and carrying weight at the abdominal region. They are usually susceptible to many diseases such as heart disease, high blood pressure, diabetes, gout and kidney disease. They have a shorter life.

Mesomorphy

The members of this group are very strong physically, having firm dense bone structure, firm muscle and strong supporting ligaments. They are more energetic and healthy. They live on an average of about as long as the best of the other types if they maintain their physical fitness and physical activities throughout life. They have strength and ruggedness and are subject to relatively few ailments unless they allow themselves to grow soft and fat from overeating and inactivity. Some of these have a tendency toward overweight in middle age.

As it was mentioned before, the body types have a genetic root that can not be altered or changed. It is fixed during the formation of the fetus. No matter what kind of diet, an endomorphic person follows, he or she will not lose more than 10-15 percent of the total body fat. If by any chance they lose more than 15 percent of total body weight, either they become sick or regain the weight back in a short time. The best advice you can give to this group is:

1. To have a balanced diet low in fat, low in calories, with more complex carbohydrates, more fruit and vegetables; so that they do not gain additional weight later in life.
2. To engage in more physical activities, to control the food calories and improve the metabolic rate.

HOW TO MEASURE YOUR WEIGHT

There are many scales that tell you what your ideal weight will be. Some of these scales are very confusing. Not everybodies frame is the same. People come in all kinds of shapes, some small, some medium and others are large.

To calculate your ideal weight you should follow the scale below.

Ideal Weight For Women

If a woman is 4'10" tall and has one of the following frames, her ideal weight would be:

Small Frame	95 Pounds
Medium Frame	105 Pounds
Large Frame	115 Pounds

If a woman is taller than 4'10", you add 3 pounds for every inch above 4'10".

For example:
A medium frame woman, 5'5" tall.

Her ideal weight would be:
>   5'5"—4'10"=7 inches
>   7"x3=21 pounds
>   21+105=126 pounds

Ideal Weight For Men
Men also come in the frames of small, medium and large.
A man with 5'2" height, his ideal weight will be:
>   Small Frame=125 pounds
>   Medium Frame=136 pounds
>   Large Frame=145 pounds

You add 4 pounds for every inch above 5'2".
For example:
For a man 5'10" with a larger frame, his ideal weight will be:
>   5'10"—5'2"=8 inches
>   8"x4=32 pounds
>   145+32=177 pounds

HOW TO MEASURE YOUR BODY FAT

There are several ways to measure your body fat.
1. Skin fold caliper
2. Underwater weighing
3. Potassium content of your muscles
4. Waist to hip ratio

The number one, two and three methods of measuring the body fat are not practical for the average person. They require professional help. But method number four is very easy to use and you may get a very good idea about your body fat content. To get an idea about your body fat use a cloth measuring tape.

1. Measure your waist about an inch above your naval.

2. Measure your hip at the widest point.

3. Divide your waist measurement by your hip measurement to find the ratio. If the ratio of waist to hip is more than 0.8, you have more fat.

Example:

If your waistline is 45 inches and your hip measurement is 50 inches, your ratio will be 45 divided by 50. It will be equal to 0.9. Your ratio is higher than 0.8, therefore your are overweight.

CHAPTER 2

DIETARY TRENDS IN THE UNITED STATES

Everybody in the United States, including children, adult men and women are facing a continuing predicament in controlling food intake and body weight. Since the Industrial Revolution the population of the United States has shifted from rural to urban areas. Most people must purchase all of their food. Even farmers, our most rural families, must purchase a substantial portion of the foods they consume. Americans have the benefit of many labor saving devices in their homes. They work fewer hours a week and have more leisure time. Leisure time for many people is comprised of less walking, more riding, watching television and eating rather than leading an active outdoor life. Greater numbers of women are working away from the home than ever before which means that there is less time available for food preparation. More people are utilizing prepared foods and eating out. With higher incomes, more meals are eaten in restaurants. The majority of workers are eating in the cafeteria at their places of work rather than carrying lunches. Children, especially teenagers, are given too much freedom in their food choices.

On the one hand, the rapid advances in technology and the improving national economy provide more varieties of food for most people. The average American family of today has a higher income and is spending more of it on food. Foods in the cupboard, the refrigerator and the freezer offer an endless variety to please every taste and palate. Colorful advertising in magazines, newspapers and television entice people to consume more and more of these manufactured products. Superb photography that illustrates recipes in homemaking magazines suggests further food temptation. Restaurants enjoy a far greater business than ever before, with emphasis being placed on a staggering quantity of food. At every social gathering, food is a very important accompaniment. Yet, the attitude of people and the pattern of living are in direct opposition to the consumption of food by the majority of people. Most people in the United States can be classified as sedentary because little physical effort is required of them whether in the office, home, school or factory. Modes of transportation used by adults and children such as cars, buses and trains have become fixtures of everyday life. Today sports have become spectator oriented with participation restricted to very skilled individuals.

It is my belief, for many people, they not only eat too much, but they do very little which brings about the physiological handicaps of obesity. The society that encourages overeating also scorns the person who is so unfortunate as to experience creeping weight gain. Even the fashion world has forgotten obese and overweight children, men and women, excluding them from fashionable society.

Increase In Chronic Illness

Today we have become a nation of processed, packaged and preserved food consumers. We spend more than 800 billion dollars per year for such items as frozen foods, snack foods, T.V. dinners as well as a tremendous amount of canned and bottled foods. By eating these foods, each of us consume every year more than four pounds of chemicals for food coloring, flavoring, stabilizing and tenderizing. With advances in technology, the amount of these artificial substances is increasing every year. Their use has been spreading to practically every food we consume. Currently, more than 3,000 chemicals are added to our food. Most of these chemicals have not been tested and proven by the Food and Drug Administration. As each year passes, more Americans become the victims of obesity, cancer and heart disease. In addition, diabetes, high blood pressure, digestive disorders, stress and mental depression are increasing. Worst of all the modern treatment of these diseases has not changed much except that we have been provided with more drugs.

America has no preventative medicine. We wait until disease progresses and then we seek treatment. Today our illnesses are chronic in nature. Most are caused by environmental factors such as poor eating habits, chemicals and lack of exercise. In spite of spending billions of dollars on the research and production of new drugs, we are still helpless to prevent any disease here in the United States. All that medical science can offer us is treatment directed at the symptoms, not at the basic cause.

The basic causes of our contemporary health problems are primarily:
1. Excessive use of additives
2. High consumption of saturated fats
2. Obesity
3. Overeating
4. Too much animal food consumption
5. Less consumption of complex carbohydrates (grain products)
6. Less consumption of fruits and vegetables
7. Eating outside the home
8. Lack of physical exercise
9. An increase in mental stress

WHY A HIGH FIBER DIET?

During this century, two very important changes have occurred in our diet. There has been a major shift in food consumption away from fruits, vegetables and whole grain products and an increase in the consumption of meat, fats and processed foods. Such major changes in our diet has caused many serious health problems such as constipation, stomach pain, diverticulitis, cancer of the colon, high cholesterol, cardiovascular disease and above all obesity. Today, a large number of Americans are having serious digestive problems such as gas, bloatedness, constipation, and diverticulitis. As consumers we spend more than three billion dollars a year for drugs, pills and laxatives to treat these problems. Television, newspapers, magazines and radio all promote a variety of drugs for quick treatment. Today the average person must take an anti-acid pill before eating and a laxative in order to go to the bathroom. Scientific studies indicate clearly that a population who consumes a high fiber diet such as fruits, vegetables and whole grain products has little problem with digestion, constipation or obesity. A high fiber diet is also recognized to contribute to a decrease in the incidence of cancer, heart disease, diabetes, digestive disorders and obesity. People who consume foods high in fat and animal products containing less fiber have a very high incidence of these diseases.

WHAT IS FIBER?

Fiber is the term used to describe indigestible carbohydrate compounds. Fiber cannot be digested by humans; therefore it is not an energy source for us. Animals do have enzymes to break down fiber and use it for energy. Fiber is found in fruits, vegetables, legumes, seeds and whole grain products. This variety of fibers have many physiological effects on human health, depending on the amount and types of fiber consumed. Not all fiber acts in the same way. Therefore it is important to consume a variety of plant foods so that we can obtain all the fiber we need. In order to obtain an adequate amount of fiber, the daily diet of each person must include fruit, green leafy vegetables, whole wheat bread, cereals, rice, potato and legumes.

LACK OF DIETARY FIBER

When a diet is high in animal foods such as beef, pork, fried foods and non-complex carbohydrates such as pie, cake, pasta, white bread and sauces, the digestive system process slows down and foods move slowly down the digestive tract. It takes a longer time to digest food and eliminate the residue (feces). During a slower movement of the foods, several important events take place in the digestive system:

1. It gives more time to the blood to absorb calories into the body. This process increases the calorie intake and eventually causes a weight gain.
2. In the small intestine, it allows the body to take more salt and more cholesterol from the digestible foods. As a result of this action, blood pressure and blood cholesterol go up.
3. Digestive residue remains for a longer period of time. A longer stay enables bacteria to feed on residue and produce toxic materials. Toxic materials damage the tissues of the colon. Eventually the tissue becomes mutagenic and then cancerous, leading to colon cancer.
4. When feces stays longer in the large intestine, it loses its water content, becoming dry and hard. This makes elimination very difficult, causing constipation.
5. Digestion of fat takes longer than digestion of protein and carbohydrate. When a diet has more fat, the digestive process slows down and the fat remains for a longer time, attracting bacterias.

Bacterias act on the fat producing a large amount of gas. Since there is no place for the gas to escape, it too remains, causing pain and bloatedness. A diet high in fiber will increase the mobility of the digestive tract. Fiber is like a sponge. It absorbs water and makes the feces soft and loose, speeding up the elimination process.

THE IMPORTANCE OF DIETARY FIBER

FIBER AS AN ANTI-CANCER AGENT

Cancer of the colon is a deadly cancer. It is the second highest killer in the United States. Fiber plays a very important role in the prevention of colon cancer. Fiber acts to decrease the transit time of waste material so that the feces will have less contact with the colon wall. Fiber also binds with bile acids. Bile acids promote cancer by irritating the colon cells and increasing cell division. Fiber also acts to prevent the production of anaerobic bacteria which feed on fecal residue, producing a toxic compound. These toxic materials are what eventually promote the development of cancer. The fiber contained in fruits and vegetables blocks the development of cancer. Cancer of the mouth, larynx, esophagus, stomach, colon, rectum and cancer of the bladder can be prevented by the consumption of fruits and vegetables which are high in fiber. A high fiber diet decreases transit time so that fecal residue has less contact with the colon walls, thus reducing contact with carcinogens. Fiber also binds bile acids and helps to block some recycling of these materials by the body. Another action of dietary fiber concerns the binding and excreting of sex hormones, testosterone and estrogen, from within the intestines. This action is very important because of the link between excessive amounts of sex hormones and certain types of cancers, especially cancer of the colon, prostrate and breast.

FIBER AS AN ANTI-CONSTIPATION AGENT

Difficult evacuation of the bowels is referred to as constipation. Constipation is caused by a slow movement of feces through the large intestine. Feces becomes dry and hard as fluids are increasingly absorbed into the blood during an extended transit time. Normal stool frequency is somewhat varied from person to person. Usually, it ranges from three to twelve times per week. The best guide for recognizing constipation is the presence of unusually hard and dry stools at infrequent intervals. Eating a high fiber diet containing fruits, vegetables and grain products is the best prevention and treatment of this condition. Dietary fiber stimulates peristalsis by helping to form a bulky stool, making it easier to evacuate without pressure. Dietary fiber acts like a sponge, absorbing water and making feces softer, allowing easier elimination.

FIBER AS AN ANTI-DIVERTICULITIS AGENT

Another disease that is associated with a low fiber diet is diverticulitis. Diverticulitis is a disease characterized by food particles becoming trapped within the pockets of the colon wall. This disease occurs in the wall of the large intestine. It is caused by the increased pressure needed to move a small and hard stool along the intestinal tract. A diet high in fiber tends to lower the pressure needed to move the stool. Fiber also acts to make the stool softer and larger.

DR. TOOSHI'S HIGH FIBER DIET

There is a good reason to believe that the abundance of calorie rich foods, especially those high in fat, are the primary reason why so many Americans are overweight. The average American consumes forty-five percent of his total calories in fat, with very little dietary fiber. As previously stated, a diet high in fat increases the transit time of the intestinal tract, causing food to remain for a longer period of time. As a result, every calorie in the food is absorbed into the blood stream. This causes weight gain. Fiber in the diet reduces transit time and increases the movement of fecal residue, resulting in fifty percent of food calories not being absorbed into the blood. This causes a weight loss.

Many people who followed my high fiber diet did not only lose weight but have told me that they feel more energetic, alert and feel very happy. Most of their problems, such as fatigue, stomach irritation due to gas, acid reflux and constipation went away. For the great majority of people, the high fiber diet provides all the essential nutrients that the human body requires for healthful living. Essential nutrients, such as carbohydrates, proteins and essential fatty acids as well as vitamins and minerals, are very important for individual well-being. The high fiber diet with its fruits, vegetables and complex carbohydrates provides a new surge of energy within a surprisingly short time. Those people who were bothered by acid reflux, gas or bloatedness were quickly relieved. A high fiber diet also releases excess fluid from the body. You will find that urination increases as water and waste are removed from your system. This, itself, helps to bring high blood pressure down and energy up. You become aware that there is greater joy in activities other than eating. You are released from such chronic illness as indigestion, constipation, shortness of breath, restricted movement and other symptoms associated with overeating and being overweight. One of the most important rewards you get from reducing weight is the surge of mental energy. Your pride in yourself, your will-power and your self confidence all will go up. You become a new person with a new philosophy and new goals facing the challenge of the future. Any goal you set becomes within your reach.

It is believed that those who successfully lose weight and change their eating habits will be successful in every aspect of life. Mental power, physical energy and the self-confidence you get from losing weight will radiate to other activities of life. The effort you make and the experience you earn will become a great asset which will turn past failure into future success.

This vital variance is why most of my dieters have been able to maintain their ideal weight year after year.

CHAPTER 3

WHY IS DR. TOOSHI'S DIET A MORE EFFECTIVE DIET?

Nutrition is a very important matter in a person's life. Our mental and physiological well-being is affected by the foods we eat. Our mood, the way we feel, act and think all are influenced by food. The food we eat can literally make our life delightful or make it a drudgery.

Nutrition is the study of how foods are digested, metabolized and turned into energy and building materials for our bodies. Nutrition can be a fascinating subject because it is about us. Unfortunately the food faddists and crackpots who have no scientific knowledge in the field of nutrition are peddling a tremendous amount of misinformation and unjustifiable claims to people through magazines, radio and television, making every thinking person confused. It is commonly agreed that a good balanced diet will help us to avoid premature aging, chronic illness and untimely death. It also gives us energy, vitality and builds resistance against environmental forces that are threatening our health. Studies conducted in both England and California evaluated 900 middle-aged men and women for a period of twelve years. The results of these studies show that coronary death rate dropped by twenty-five percent for those who ate a diet containing fruits, vegetables and high fiber foods.

A close association between cancer and heart disease and a low fiber diet was reported by the Center for Disease Control in Atlanta, Georgia. Another study found that women who ate few fruits and vegetables (low fiber) had twenty-five percent more incidence of breast cancer than women who had more fruits and vegetables in their diets. Today people are told that you must have a balanced diet. We know that there are so many diets from which to choose. All of these diets are deficient in some basic nutrients. Some of these diets are high carbohydrate diets, high protein diets, liquid protein diets, chocolate food diets, grapefruit diets, diet pills and frozen food diets. These diets can not provide the essential nutrients that our body needs to function at its best. Our body needs carbohydrates to produce energy for physical and mental work, protein to build and maintain our body, fat to manufacture hormones, enzymes and protection against radiation. In addition, fiber, vitamins and minerals to digest, metabolize and anabolize the food we eat must be consumed. The above mentioned foods are essential to build the immune system so that we are protected against cancer, heart disease and tumors.

Dr. Tooshi's Diet is made up from natural carbohydrates, proteins, unsaturated fats, vegetables, fruits and fiber. His diet not only provides all essential ingredients to your body but it also helps you to lose weight and improve your health and well-being. His diet is easy to follow. You need not worry about weighing or measuring foods. Your breakfast, lunch and dinner for each day has been planned for you. You need do nothing; just follow the diet. There is also an excellent maintenance diet which has been organized for you to follow once you achieve your desired weight.

CASE STUDIES

CASE 1
Jean was a twenty-five year old attractive woman, who had a serious problem with gas and gas related pain. For a few years she was taking medication and had visited several doctors. She had taken many G.I. tests. They all came back negative. She was told there was nothing wrong with her. She was also advised not to eat any fruits and vegetables. After following her doctors advice, still the pain did not go away. Finally, her friend advised her to see me. I introduced her to my high fiber diet and within two days the gas was gone and the pain disappeared.

CASE 2
Linda had, for many years, a serious dermatological problem. Since she was fourteen years of age, she had visited many doctors and took several different medications and topical creams. None had helped her. Her face and back were covered with pimples. Because of her appearance she was very shy and had little self-confidence. After I introduced her to my high fiber diet, I advised her not to use any make-up or creams. Within one month her face cleared up and she had no more skin problems. Six months later she called me and thanked me for my help.

CASE 3
Ed was a sixty-seven year old man with diabetes, high cholesterol, high blood pressure and was forty-five pounds overweight. After putting him on my high fiber diet for almost three months, his blood pressure dropped from 160 to 130 systolic, his cholesterol dropped 25 points and his blood sugar became normal without taking medication.

CASE 4
Barbara, an assistant manager of a bank, had no energy especially early in the morning and late evenings. She had visited several doctors

and had been taking medications for almost eight months. None of the medications were helping her. I planned a high fiber diet and prescribed some vitamins. Within a few days she was feeling energetic, sleeping well and feeling good.

CASE 5
Norma, a school teacher, complained of chest pain after eating. She told me that several times, in the middle of the night, she had to go to the emergency room because of severe chest pain. She felt that she might be getting a heart attack. However, there was nothing wrong with her heart. The doctor told her that the pain might be from her stomach. She was referred to me. She followed my high fiber diet and within two to three days she had no pain at all.

CASE 6
Nancy, a registered nurse, was complaining about fatigue and being light-headed. She had problems sleeping. During the day she was feeling tired and hungry. She felt tense and irritable all day long. From the information that she provided to me, I realized that she has low blood sugar. I put her on my hypoglycemic diet and within a week she was feeling good. She had no problem sleeping.

CASE 7
Walter, a retired railroad man, 56 years old, had high cholesterol, high blood pressure and very high triglycerides of 450 Mg/cc. He was on many medications for more than seven years. He was currently taking medication for high cholesterol and high blood pressure when I met him. I put him on my high fiber diet. After following the diet for one month, his cholesterol dropped 32 points, his triglycerides dropped 265 points and his blood pressure dropped to 126/84. He was suddenly energetic and felt good again. He no longer needed medication.

CASE 8
Jackie was a 42 year old housewife who had high blood pressure and constant headaches. She was taking high blood pressure pills for six years. She told me she feels like an old woman. After following my high fiber diet, her blood pressure dropped to a normal level and the headaches were gone. She lost 22 pounds and her doctor took her off the blood pressure pills. She said to me "I feel like a new person".

CASE 9
Herman, at 55 years of age, weighed 225 pounds and had diabetes. He was taking medication for diabetes for more than three years and his blood pressure was 164/106 at the start of the diet program. Within one week, his blood sugar dropped 46 points and within one month both his blood sugar and blood pressure were at normal ranges without medication. He lost 35 pounds.

CASE 10
M.S., a male of 5'10", weighing 381 pounds, said he was determined to take off 150 pounds. He had a problem of breathing and felt extremely tired. In addition he had gout and high blood pressure. Although he was only 38 years old, he said he felt like an old man. While following my diet plan, he went down to 260 pounds over a period of eight months. His blood pressure dropped to a normal 124/80 and his gout disappeared with his big weight loss. He commented to me "I feel like a new man".

CASE 11
M.W., a teacher at 5'3" and weighing 212 pounds, said that she tried every diet to lose weight more than once without any success. Each time she would lose a few pounds, she would gain it right back. By following my diet, she lost 76 pounds and kept it off. When she visited me almost ten years later, she told me that this was the first

time that she has maintained her weight so well without gaining it back. She told me "your diet changed my life. It gave me a new outlook".

CASE 12
E.W., a teacher at 5'11", weighing 228 pounds instead of his ideal weight of 190 pounds, had high blood pressure and was taking medication to keep it under control. During the first month on my diet he lost 23 pounds and his blood pressure dropped to 122/80. During the second month he dropped 15 more pounds. He was very proud of himself.

CASE 13
P.G., a woman at 5'10", weighing 186 pounds, told me that she felt tired and could not sleep at night. I put her on my high fiber diet. Within two weeks she lost 14 pounds. She got her energy back and had no problems sleeping through the night. Within two months, she lost 36 pounds. I planned a maintenance diet for her. She attained her ideal weigh of 135 pounds and has successfully maintained it for many years.

M.B.
Bayonne, New Jersey 07002
March 12, 1998

Dear Dr. Tooshi,
Just wanted to thank you for all the help and moral support in the last month. I could not have lost the 15 pounds without you. Unfortunately, my financial obligation for school registration and tuition for the children has strapped me for the time being.
I promise to continue where we left off and follow your diet plan so that I can lose 15 more pounds to meet my goal. I even purchased a

country music aerobic video that I am doing with my daughter..I will keep in touch and thank you for getting me started.

M.B.

CHAPTER 4

DR. TOOSHI'S DIET PROGRAMS

PROGRAM ONE
Lose Up To 5 Pounds In One Week

PROGRAM TWO
Lose Up To 10 Pounds In Two—Three Weeks

PROGRAM THREE
Lose Up To 20 Pounds In Four—Six Weeks

PROGRAM FOUR
Lose More Than 20 Pounds

DIET PLAN ONE:
Lose Up To 5 Pounds In One Week

This diet has been planned for those who wish to attend weddings, class reunions and birthday parties; or if your favorite clothing or jeans are a little tighter and you just don't feel comfortable in them. This is the diet for you. Everything has been organized in such a way that it will be very easy for you to lose weight and achieve your goal within a few days. The breakfast, lunch and dinner for each day indicates what you should eat. It is also a very balanced diet. It has carbohydrates for energy, protein for growth, fat for protection of the hair and skin, and fruits and vegetables for vitamin and mineral sources. You have the option to select any breakfast, lunch or dinner from the list. To be sure you know how much weight you are losing, you should check your weight every day when you get up in the morning.

When you achieve your weight goal, you should follow the maintenance diet. You will keep your weight under control for many years for a healthier life.

How To Measure Your Weight

It is very important that you know how to measure your body weight correctly. You need to know how much weight you are losing as you follow your diet. There are a few things you need to know. First, you will need a reliable scale. Next, you should know how to measure the reliability of your scale.

How To Measure The Reliability Of Your Scale
1. Your scale is balanced when you move it to zero. If it is not balanced, the scale is not reliable.
2. Step on the scale. Look at your weight. Record it.

3. Step off the scale. Look to see if it returns to zero. If the scale does not return to zero, the scale is no good.

4. If the scale does return to zero after stepping off, then step on again and look at your weight. If the two measurements are the same, then your scale is reliable.

DIET PLAN ONE:
LOSE UP TO 5 POUNDS IN ONE WEEK

(SELECT ONE OF THE FOLLOWING FOR BREAKFAST, LUNCH AND DINNER)

BREAKFAST:
1. A fruit
2. A slice of whole wheat or rye bread with a teaspoon of jam
LUNCH:
1. Salad with turkey
2. Salad with an egg
3. Two fruits
DINNER:
1. Chicken cutlet
2. Fish La Chanta
3. Baked Flounder
4. Chicken La Shabo
A fruit late at night if desired.
Helpful Hints:
All dinner recipes can be found in the "Recipes Chapter" at the end of the book.

Do not eat the same food every day. Vary your choices.

Do not eat any one item more than two times per week.

If the above choices do not satisfy your needs or preferences, you may select from the following items:

BREAKFAST:

A fruit, ½ grapefruit, oatmeal with a little low fat milk, a slice of toast with a teaspoon of jam, a hard boiled egg, ½ cantaloupe, an English muffin with a teaspoon of jam, a bagel with a teaspoon of jam.

LUNCH:

Salad with turkey, fruit salad

DINNER:

Lean steak with salad, grilled chicken with salad or vegetables, fish with steamed vegetables.

WHAT YOU SHOULD DRINK

Water is the most versatile medium for all kinds of chemical reactions in the body. Without water, life processes would cease in a matter of days. We require, on average, two quarts of water per day and it must be replenished daily because the body can not store water well. A person should drink 5 to 6 glasses of water daily in order to create a suitable environment so that the physiological activities of the body can be carried on smoothly.

Water performs many functions in the body. Some major functions of water are:

A) It lubricates joints

B) Transports nutrients, minerals, vitamins and other substances throughout the body

C) Water controls body temperature

D) It removes waste materials out of the body

E) Water prevents constipation and cancer by softening the stool and eliminating it

F) Water prevents the blood from becoming thicker, preventing clotting

G) Water prevents dehydration of the body tissues

Therefore, it is important for us to take at least 5 to 6 glasses of fluid per day. The best fluid is water itself, but you can also drink the following beverages:

1. Homemade ice tea with lemon and/or an artificial sweetener (aspartame).
2. Water with lemon and/or artificial sweetener
3. Hot tea with lemon and/or artificial sweetener
4. Coffee with one percent milk and/or artificial sweetener

Note: You should avoid the following:

1. Sodas
2. Punch drinks
3. Canned, jarred, and bottled foods
4. Precooked foods

These foods and drinks are very high in salt and additives. They increase blood pressure, retain water, aggravate arthritis and may cause cancer.

SEASONINGS

Use of seasoning to spice up your food provides you with taste and flavor. It also helps you to enjoy your foods. Chopped parsley and chives add a very tasty touch to your chicken and vegetables. This fresh flavor is easy to achieve since parsley and chives are sold in small packages in many food stores. Oregano, lemon, pepper, hot fresh pepper or other flavorful Italian seasonings and spices all enhance plain green beans and other vegetables. Wedges of lemon, herbs, and vinegar also provide great satisfaction. There are perhaps a hundred tasty relishes to improve the flavor of your food; but you must use them in moderation and use your judgement.

EATING OUT

If you are planning to eat out while following this diet, you can select from any one of the following:

BREAKFAST:
A fruit, any one fruit
A bagel with jam
Oatmeal

LUNCH:
Salad with turkey
Salad with an egg
A bagel with jam
Fruit salad

DINNER:
Turkey sandwich
Lean steak with salad
Grilled chicken with salad
Grilled fish with vegetables
Steamed shrimp with steamed vegetables

DIET PLAN TWO
LOSE UP TO 10 POUNDS IN 3 WEEKS

This diet has been planned for those who wish to attend up-coming weddings, class reunions, a special function or for those feeling tired, lacking energy and generally not feeling good about themselves. Everything has been organized in such a way that it will be very easy for you to follow and achieve your goal. The breakfast, lunch and dinner menus for each day indicate what you should eat. This diet is also a very well-balanced diet. It has carbohydrates for energy, protein for growth, fat for protection of hair and skin, as well as fruits and vegetables as sources of vitamins and minerals.

You have the option to select any breakfast, lunch and dinner from the list as you wish. To be sure how much weight you are losing, you should check your weight daily when you get up in the morning before eating breakfast. After you achieve your goal, you should follow the maintenance diet I have provided later in the book. You will keep your weight under control for many years for a healthier life.

DIET PLAN TWO
WEEK 1

Select any one of the Breakfast, Lunch and Dinners. Do not eat any one item more than twice in one week.

BREAKFAST:

1. Fruit
2. Toast with a teaspoon of jam

LUNCH:

1. Salad with turkey
2. Salad with an egg
3. Salad with tuna fish

DINNER:

1. Chicken Cutlet
2. Fish La Chanta
3. Tooshi's Dinner

A fruit or salad at night if desired

NOTE: See salad dressing recipe

DRINKS: Coffee, tea or water. No soda.

WEEK 2

BREAKFAST:
1. Oatmeal
2. An English muffin
3. A hard boiled egg

LUNCH:
1. Plain, low-fat yogurt with a fruit
2. An egg with a fruit
3. A glass of low-fat milk with a fruit

DINNER:
1. Tooshi's Delight
2. Shrimp Dinner
3. Lean steak with salad

A fruit or salad at night

WEEK 3

BREAKFAST:
1. A banana
2. ½ cantaloupe
3. Toast with a teaspoon of jam

LUNCH:
1. An egg with a fruit
2. Tuna with tomato and chopped onion
3. Salad with turkey

DINNER:
1. Baked Flounder
2. Egg Omelet
3. Chicken La Shabo

A fruit or slice of toast at night

EATING OUT

DINNER:
You may select any of the following items.
1. Lean steak with salad
2. Grilled chicken with salad or vegetables
3. Fish with steamed vegetables
4. Turkey sandwich

LUNCH:
1. Salad with turkey
2. Fruit salad

BREAKFAST:
1. ½ grapefruit
2. A fruit
3. A toast with teaspoon of jam

DRINKS:
1. Coffee, tea or water
2. Homemade ice tea with lemon and/or artificial sweetener
3. Water with lemon and/or artificial sweetener
4. Hot tea with lemon and/or artificial sweetener
5. Coffee with 1% milk and/or artificial sweetener

NOTE: you should avoid the following items.
1. Soda
2. Punch
3. Canned, jarred and bottled foods
4. Precooked foods

These foods and drinks are very high in salt and chemical additives.

They increase blood pressure, retain water, aggravate arthritis and may cause cancer.

SEASONINGS: Use of seasonings to spice up your food provides you with taste and flavor. You enjoy your food more when you select spices that enhance the flavor. Be careful and use spices in moderation. Avoid using spices that contain salt as an ingredient.

SNACKS: You can select any one of the following snack foods.

1. Baby carrots	(3 oz)
2. Fresh fruit	(One)
3. Fig bar	(One)
4. Graham crackers	(.5 oz or two crackers)
5. Rice cake	(Two)
6. Air-popped popcorn	(1 cup, popped)
7. Animal crackers	(.5 oz or five crackers)
8. Ginger snaps	(.5 oz or three cookies)
9. Saltines	(Five crackers)
10. Whole wheat crackers	(.5 oz or three crackers)

DIET PLAN THREE:
LOSE UP TO 20 POUNDS IN SIX WEEKS

According to statistics, forty-five percent of people in America are overweight. Most of these people are 20 pounds above the normal body weight. These statistics also show that most people in this group gained weight after the age of twenty-five. They had normal body weight between the ages eighteen to twenty. The reasons responsible for such weight gain are:

A) Less physical activity

B) Increased social activity (attending more social functions)

C) Declining metabolism as a result of aging

As people get older, body cells become less active and do not utilize energy as they used to. Therefore, as a result of aging, excessive calorie intake is stored in the body as fat. Diet Plan Three has been organized for people in this group. The breakfast, lunch and dinner for each day indicates what you will be eating. This diet is a balanced diet. It has carbohydrates for energy, protein for growth, fat for protection of hair and skin, and fruits and vegetables as sources of vitamins and minerals. You have the option to select any breakfast, lunch or dinner from the list as you wish.

DIET PLAN 3
WEEK 1

Select any one of the breakfasts, lunches or dinners. Do not select any one item more than twice per week.

BREAKFAST:
1. A fruit
2. A slice of toast with a teaspoon of jam

LUNCH:
1. Salad with turkey
2. Salad with an egg
3. Salad with tuna fish

DINNER:
1. Chicken cutlet
2. Fish La Chanta
3. Tooshi's Dinner
A fruit or small salad at night if desired.
NOTE: See salad dressing recipe
DRINKS:
1. Coffee, tea or water
2. No sodas

WEEK 2

BREAKFAST:
1. Oatmeal
2. An English muffin
3. A hard boiled egg

LUNCH:
1. Plain, low-fat yogurt with a fruit
2. An egg with a fruit
3. A glass of low-fat milk with a fruit
DINNER:
1. Tooshi's Delight
2. Shrimp Dinner
3. Lean steak with salad
A fruit or salad at night if desired

WEEK 3

BREAKFAST:
1. A banana
2. ½ cantaloupe
3. Toast with a teaspoon of jam
LUNCH:
1. An egg with a fruit
2. Tuna with tomato and chopped onion
3. Salad with turkey
DINNER:
1. Baked Flounder
2. Egg Omelet
3. Chicken La Shabo
A fruit or slice of toast at night if desired

WEEK 4

BREAKFAST:
1. An egg
2. A fruit
3. Toast with jam

LUNCH:
1. A glass of milk with a banana
2. An egg with a fruit
3. Salad with tuna
4. Salad with a fruit

DINNER:
1. Hamburger with lettuce, tomato, onion and two slices toast
2. Fish La Chanta
3. Chicken Cutlet
4. Egg Omelet

WEEK 5

BREAKFAST:
1. An English muffin with jam
2. Oatmeal
3. A banana
4. A hard boiled egg

LUNCH:
1. Yogurt with a fruit
2. Toast with tomato and a slice of Alpine Lace cheese
3. Toast with tomato and a slice of turkey

DINNER:
1. Lean steak with salad
2. Tooshi's Dinner
3. Vegetarian Dinner
4. Shrimp Salad
5. Turkey sandwich

WEEK 6

BREAKFAST:
1. Oatmeal
2. Toast with jam
3. ½ grapefruit

LUNCH:
1. Toast with a slice of cheese and tomato
2. Two slices of toast with sliced tomato (tomato sandwich)
3. ½ cantaloupe with two tablespoons of cottage cheese
DINNER:
1. Lamb chop with salad or vegetables
2. Stuffed Flounder
3. Stuffed Peppers
A fruit at night if desired

EATING OUT

DINNER:
You may order from the following items.
1. Lean steak with salad
2. Grilled chicken with salad or vegetables
3. Fish with steamed vegetables
4. Turkey sandwich
LUNCH:
1. Salad with turkey
2. Fruit salad
BREAKFAST:
1. ½ grapefruit
2. A fruit
3. An egg with a slice of toast

DRINKS: Coffee, tea or water. Add 1% low-fat milk, lemon or artificial sweetener only.
   SNACKS: You may select any one of the following items to snack on.

Baby carrots	(3 oz)
Air-popped popcorn	(1 cup, popped)
Fresh fruit	(One)
Animal crackers	(.5 oz /five crackers)
Fig bar	(One)

Ginger snaps	(.5 oz /three cookies)
Graham crackers	(.5oz/two crackers)
Saltines	(Five crackers)
Rice cakes	(Two)
Whole wheat crackers	(.5 oz/three crackers)

DIET PLAN 4:
LOSE MORE THAN 20 POUNDS

People who need to lose more than twenty pounds may follow Diet Plan 4. Today, there are a variety of diets on the market for people who are overweight. Diets ranging from grapefruit diets to protein shakes, medications, pills, chocolate shakes and liquid diets are available; but so far none of these diets have helped people to lose weight permanently. Any weight that people lose through the use of these diets is water, not fat. As soon as they go off these diets they gain the weight back. The use of such diets produce dehydration, which causes fatigue and may consequently lead to heart attack. Pills and drugs, too, have serious side effects. They may cause brain damage and produce tumors of the brain. The only safe way to lose weight is through balanced nutrition and reduced calories. Such a diet must include carbohydrates, proteins, fruits and vegetables. Diet Program 4 is a nutritionally perfect diet. It helps you to lose weight, improve your health, increase your energy and vitalize your day.

Start your diet with Diet Plan 2 "Lose 10 Pounds in Three Weeks", then go to Diet Plan 3 "Lose 20 Pounds in Six Weeks". After that you follow Diet Plan 4 "Lose More Than 20 Pounds". Everything has been organized in such a way that it is easy to lose weight and achieve your goal. The breakfast, lunch and dinners for each day indicate what you should eat. The entire diet program is well-balanced and easy to follow. Make sure that you do not choose each breakfast, lunch and dinner more than twice a week.

DIET PLAN 4

BREAKFAST:
1. A fruit, any kind
2. Oatmeal (one serving) with or without milk
3. An English muffin with a teaspoon of jam
4. A slice of toast with a slice of Alpine Lace cheese
5. An egg
6. A bagel with a teaspoon of jam
7. A slice of toast with a teaspoon of jam
8. ½ cantaloupe
9. ½ grapefruit

LUNCH:
1. An egg with a fruit
2. An egg with a slice of toast and tomato
3. A slice of cheese with toast and tomato
4. A slice of turkey with toast and tomato
5. A glass of milk with a banana
6. A bagel with a teaspoon of jam
7. Cottage cheese (3 tbsp.) Low-fat with a fruit
8. Salad with turkey
9. Salad with tuna
10. Salad with an egg
11. Sardines with salad
12. Salad with a fruit
13. Salad with a slice of cheese
14. Tuna with chopped onion and tomato
15. Two fruits
16. Tomato sandwich (two slices toast with tomato)

17. Yogurt, low-fat, with a fruit
18. Fruit Salad (any three fruits)

DINNERS:

1. Baked Flounder
2. Chicken Cutlet
3. Chicken La Shabo
4. Egg Omelet
5. Fish La Chanta
6. Grilled Chicken with Salad
7. Lean Steak with Salad
8. Pasta with Tooshi's Sauce
9. Rice with Tooshi's Sauce
10. Shrimp Dinner
11. Tooshi's Dinner
12. Turkey Sandwich
13. Vegetarian Dinner
14. Oriental Supreme

EATING OUT:

Dinner:
You may order from the following items.
1. Lean steak with a salad
2. Grilled chicken with salad or vegetables
3. Fish with steamed vegetables
4. Turkey sandwich

Lunch:
1. Salad with turkey
2. Fruit salad

Breakfast:
1. ½ grapefruit
2. A fruit
3. A slice of toast with a teaspoon of jam

BEVERAGES:

Coffee, tea or water
You may add lemon, low-fat milk or artificial sweetener.

SNACKS:

1. Baby carrots	(3 oz.)
2. Fresh fruit	(One)
3. Fig Bar	(One)
4. Graham crackers	(.5 oz or two crackers)
5. Rice cakes	(Two)
6. Air-popped popcorn	(1 cup, popped)
7. Animal crackers	(.5 oz. or five crackers)
8. Ginger snaps	(.5 oz. or three cookies)
9. Saltines	(Five)
10. Whole wheat crackers	(.5 oz. or three crackers)

CHAPTER 5

THE CHARACTERISTICS OF A SOUND MAINTENANCE DIET

Today, consumers pour more than 33 billion dollars into the diet industry. It is a business that has been growing day by day and year by year since the mid-nineteen seventies. The diet industries, too, are spending a lot of money to promote their products. Diet pills, protein shakes, herbs, candy bars, frozen foods and vitamin supplements are some of the products available to weight conscious individuals. If these products had a real effect on losing weight then we would not have a growing number of overweight people in the United States. Today almost 66 percent of the population are overweight and more than 25 percent of these people are obese. It is important to understand that the goal of these diet industries is not to help people to lose weight, but to make money. Consumers must educate themselves to understand that you cannot get rid of unwanted weight by using pills, shakes, herbs, vitamins or packaged foods. It is not healthy or effective to curb your appetite with chemicals or food substitutes. You will be jeopardizing your health and increasing your risk for cancer, gall stones, kidney stones and circulatory problems. The best approach to losing weight must consider the following:

1. Reducing food intake
2. Changing your eating habits

3. Selecting foods that are naturally low in fat and low in calorie
4. Eating more fruits and vegetables
5. Engaging more in daily physical activities

A good maintenance diet must contain the following characteristics:

1. Provide a well balanced diet, including fruits, vegetables and grain products
2. Contain vitamins, minerals and essential nutrients
3. The ability to dine out and select nutritional foods

In planning my diet I have given much consideration to the following:

1. To help you to lose weight and to keeping it off
2. Providing sufficient essential nutrients
3. Reducing the chances of getting chronic diseases such as high blood pressure, cancer and heart disease
4. Planning the diet around familiar, available and appetizing foods
5. Providing a natural diet without additives

THE MAINTENANCE DIET

Once you have achieved your weight loss goal and want to maintain your weight, you will need to follow the Maintenance Diet. You may select any one of the food items in each category. Do not eat the same item more than three times per week. You need to maintain a variety of foods in your diet in order to get proper nutrition.

BREAKFAST:

1. Two eggs (boiled or poached) with two slices of toast
2. A bagel with a slice of low-fat cheese
3. Cereal with 1% milk and raisins or banana
4. ½ cantaloupe
5. An English muffin with jam or a slice of cheese
6. Fruit salad

LUNCH:

1. Turkey sandwich with lettuce and tomato
2. Tuna sandwich with lettuce and tomato

3. Cheese sandwich with lettuce and tomato

4. Egg sandwich with lettuce and tomato

5. Plain, low-fat yogurt with a fruit

6. Salad with turkey

7. Shrimp Salad

8. A bagel with a slice of cheese

9. Two fruits with a hard boiled egg

10. Fruit salad

DINNER:

1. Chicken cutlet with potato

2. Fish La Chanta with rice

3. Tooshi's Dinner with rice

4. Shrimp Dinner with rice or potato

5. Egg Omelet with rice or pasta

6. Lean steak with potato and salad

SOCIAL EVENTS

When you are invited to a social event, you find yourself among a tremendous variety of foods and drinks which are very high in salt and fat. Because of the effects of the social environment and social pressure, you find it difficult to resist eating or tasting many of these foods. The best way to solve this problem is to control your appetite. You will have more appetite and you will eat more food if you have missed one meal prior to attending a social event. This is a very important factor that needs to be taken into consideration. Most people gain two to five pounds after a social event. Most of the weight gain is not fat, but water that you are retaining. And, most party foods have a high salt content and you already know that salt retains water in the body.

HOW TO DEAL WITH A SOCIAL EVENT

You can have a good time at a party and at the same time not gain weight. Just follow a simple guideline.

1. Do not miss any of your meals. If you are planning to attend a party at night and having your dinner there, make sure that you do not skip your lunch. Many people will avoid eating lunch trying to save calories, however by the time they arrive to the party they are hungry and actually consume more food.

2. Do not consume too much of any one food. If the meal is buffet style, pick up a plate and select a tablespoon of all the things you like. This will satisfy your appetite and desire to taste a variety of foods.

3. Be careful about the beverages you consume. Most are high in salt and calories. Drink water with ice or lemon. Limit alcoholic beverages to one glass of wine or one cocktail and drink it slowly.

4. Another way to reduce calorie intake is to circulate and talk to people. Usually people who talk more, eat less.

5. Check your weight in the morning after the party.

If you gained weight, follow this one day diet:

ONE-DAY DIET AFTER A PARTY

BREAKFAST:
1. A fruit

LUNCH: (select one)
1. Two fruits
2. An egg with a fruit
3. Salad

DINNER: (select one)
1. Chicken Cutlet
2. Fish La Chanta
3. Egg Omelet
4. Shrimp Dinner

EATING OUT

Today, eating out has become a common event among Americans. Busy schedules with both husband and wife working leave little time to cook and prepare foods at home. Commercial advertising, television, radio and newspapers invite people to eat out. Many restaurants and eateries are competing to attract more customers by offering more food for less money. These eating establishments are aware that Americans love large portions, high in fat and salt. Take, for example, Chinese food. Most people like Chinese food because of the taste. Chinese kitchens add more salt and fat to the foods they offer their American customers, while the Chinese themselves eat a lot of vegetables with plain rice and almost no salt or fat.

EATING OUT—SITTING STYLE:

In this setting you are given a full course meal.
A) Bread and butter
B) Soup
C) Salad
D) Main Course
E) Dessert

The bread and butter are basically empty calories, having no nutritional values. They contain between 300 to 500 calories. Soup served at restaurants is made up from beef or chicken extraction. If you have a hypertension and water retention problem then you will have a big problem if you eat the soup. The average serving of soup contains 250 to 300 calories. Concerning the salad, there is no benefit eating salad at night. Salad is good during lunch, but with its ingredients and dressing will add 200 to 300 additional calories to your evening meal. The main course usually consists of a beef, chicken or seafood dish, vegetables or salad, and rice, potato or pasta. A main course meal can contain between 500 to 600 calories. The main course is followed by dessert.

In America, most desserts consist of cakes, pies or pastries. Desserts can contain anywhere from 250 to 400 calories. Therefore, the total caloric content of a full course sit-down dinner could be:

Bread and butter	400—600 calories
Soup	250—400 calories
Salad	200—250 calories
Main Course	500—600 calories
Dessert	300—400 calories

The total calories for a typical dinner out contain between 1,650 to 2,250 calories. You can see, then, how the cumulative effect of eating out can cause weight gain. You can enjoy a dinner out and prevent weight gain if you just limit yourself to the main course. Eating larger amounts of food will increase the size of the stomach, which is associated with higher appetite. By reducing the size of your dinner, you will help to shrink the size of your stomach and lower your appetite.

DINNER OUT—BUFFET STYLE:

If you are dining out and it is a buffet style dinner, you should have no problem enjoying the foods and controlling your weight. The first thing you need to do is to get a plate and select a tablespoon of all the foods you like. Second, try to avoid fried foods and foods high in salt. Remember not to overload your stomach.

HOW TO CONTROL SPECIAL EVENTS:

Special events are a very important part of life. They provide us with social accessibility, fun and relaxation. Social events can alleviate stress and mental fatigue. They are part of our cultural lives. We all participate in them and most of us enjoy them. But when we go overboard and eat and drink too much we face several problems the next day. Some of these problems could be acid stomach, bloatedness and weight gain. Sometimes we find ourselves with a 4 to 8 pound weight gain, making us very uncomfortable. But do not panic, help is underway. For my readers who may face this problem, I have planned a one day diet that works magic.

You should know that the weight gained after a party is not all fat; it is mostly water. The food you had eaten was very high in salt. It is the salt that is holding the water in your body. This one day diet will work like magic and release the water right away.

The only thing you have to do is follow it for just one day.

ONE DAY DIET

BREAKFAST:
A fruit

LUNCH: (select one)
An egg with a fruit
Two fruits
A salad

DINNER:
Fish La Chanta
Chicken Cutlet
Steak with salad

DRINKS: Water, tea, coffee
NO: Soda, juice or alcoholic beverages

CHAPTER 6

DR. TOOSHI'S EXERCISE PROGRAM

WHY SHOULD YOU EXERCISE ?

The purpose of life in primitive culture was to obtain food, secure shelter and provide protection. To achieve these objectives, man had to swim rivers, chase animals, climb trees and build shelters. These daily activities kept him healthy and physically active throughout his life. Even American pioneers who settled in the new land were engaged in a constant hand to hand combat with their environment. They had a difficult time surviving. All their daily chores had to be done manually. With no technological aids, they built homes and railroads, cultivated land and raised cattle.

We have the same kind of body as that created for ancient man, a body that was designed for physical activity. However, the Industrial Revolution changed mans way of life. It brought machines which have virtually eliminated the necessity of walking, running, lifting and climbing. In homes, factories and even on farms, machines now supply the power for most jobs.

Today the ordinary tasks of daily living no longer provide adequate physical activity to maintain and develop a healthy cardiovascular system and a normal body weight. Inactivity, together with poor eating habits have resulted in a critical health problem. Today the death rate from heart disease among the middle-aged population continues to climb at an alarming rate. Physiologically, male adults in their thirties are a mess. A man climbing a few flights of stairs is gasping for his breath. A commuter, sprinting to catch the train is ready to drop in his tracks, and a day of housework leaves a typical person exhausted.

We are the most sports minded of all nations. We spend billions of dollars to purchase sports equipment and to build sports arenas to accommodate a handful of college and professional athletes; then, we sit and watch them play. Today the rapid rise in professional sports on television has allowed the American people to become armchair athletes, complete with all the game knowledge and techniques any champion athlete would require. But they are experts orally, of course, and usually from a reclining chair. Most of the living room athletes would likely suffer a heart attack with their first effort to play the real game.

Weekend exercise is a familiar activity to many people. They spend five days a week at a sedentary desk job that requires almost no physical effort. When Saturday and Sunday come around, they play tennis, golf or sometimes shovel heavy snow. It never occurs to them that sudden exertion after prolonged periods of inactivity makes them a prime candidate for a heart attack. During the last thirty years, the number of physically unfit people has been increasing drastically.

HOW HARD SHOULD YOU EXERCISE ?

The ability of the body to withstand the stresses set up by physical exercise depends mainly on the ability of the cardiovascular system to supply and utilize oxygen, and to dispose of the rapidly mounting concentration of lactic acid and carbon dioxide. Sedentary people tend to have a very low cardiovascular capacity and they are unable to deliver an adequate amount of oxygen to the working muscles. Therefore, the intensity of exercise for such individuals should be adjusted to the degree of their physical conditions. Today, the pulse rate is used as a basis for determining the intensity of exercise, regardless of the individual level of physical fitness, age, sex and body weight. The intensity of exercise should be about seventy percent of a person's maximum pulse rate. This pulse rate is called training pulse rate or TPR.

CALCULATION OF THE TRAINING PULSE RATE

To obtain the training pulse rate, follow these steps:
1. Subtract your age from 220. You will get your maximum pulse rate.
1. Subtract your age from 220. You will get your maximum pulse rate.
    220—Age=Maximum Pulse Rate
2. Find 70% of your maximum pulse rate. This will give you your training pulse rate.
    Maximum Pulse Rate x 70=Training Pulse Rate
    100

Example:

A person, age 30.
    220-30=190 Maximum Pulse Rate
    190x70=133 Exercise Pulse Rate
    100

You should not let your pulse rate go beyond your exercise pulse rate during physical activity.

HOW MUCH AND HOW OFTEN SHOULD YOU EXERCISE?

Regular physical exercise is essential to good health. No one can obtain a satisfactory level of cardiovascular fitness and maintain a good body weight by exercising once a week or with a weekend of playing golf or tennis. Statistical studies have indicated that once a week exercise is harmful and actually dangerous. Once a week exercise patterns place a greater pressure on the cardiac muscle and require that a larger amount of oxygen be delivered to the working muscles. Since the cardiovascular systems of sedentary people are not adjusted to strenuous exercise and have little capacity to deliver larger amounts of oxygen to the body, damage may result to the heart or cause a heart attack. We have heard many instances of people who have died as a result of exercising, working in the garden, shoveling snow or jogging. According to research, one should exercise at least three times a week in order to improve his health. Of course, one who exercises everyday will benefit more than those who exercise three times a week.

HOW MUCH EXERCISE IS BENEFICIAL ?

The length of an exercise program is of the utmost importance in achieving a good cardiovascular fitness. An exercise session should last between twenty to thirty minutes. This does not include warm-up time. Exercise programs lasting less than twenty minutes do not produce a beneficial effect on the cardiac muscle. In other words, it cannot lower blood pressure, blood cholesterol, reduce body weight or prevent heart disease.

THE STATIONARY BICYCLE

Many people today avoid participating in any type of physical exercise due to a lack of skill, space, difficulty in finding available facilities or the time to exercise on a regular basis. The stationary bicycle is the answer to these excuses and is considered one of the best methods of exercising to improve the cardiovascular system for the following reasons:

1. It can be worked into any daily schedule
2. It does not require instruction or special skills
3. It can be set up anywhere in a home or office environment
4. There are no seasonal or weather restrictions

5. Anyone, regardless of fitness level, can exercise on the bicycle
6. Bicycle exercise requires oxygen utilization, vital for a healthy cardiovascular system
7. It produces maximum cardiovascular benefit in a short period of time
8. Calories burnt up in pedaling can produce a major weight loss

HOW TO USE THE STATIONARY BICYCLE

The user of a stationary bicycle should know how to measure and regulate speed as well as resistance. Intensity of resistance can be mechanically increased by either tightening a strap which applies friction to the flywheel or by adjusting a knob or dial mechanism. The speed of pedaling is regulated by a metronome on the bicycle at a rate of fifty to sixty revolutions per minute.

OPERATION

To avoid overexertion, first find your individual training resistance by finding your Training Pulse Rate. Begin by pedaling for three minutes at a zero workload (resistance) and at a speed of fifty to sixty revolutions per minute. Then, increase the workload every three minutes until your pulse rate is equal to your training pulse rate. At this point, stop pedaling and record the resistance. This is your training resistance. Now you can set up a reasonable training schedule to follow to improve your condition.

When you are able to ride the bicycle 25 to 30 minutes at your training workload (resistance), you may increase your workload. Any workload increase must be based on your Training Pulse Rate. Conditioning lowers the TPR so that each month you should increase your workload until it raises your pulse rate to the level of your Training Pulse Rate.

A PROGRESSIVE TRAINING PROGRAM FOR THE STATIONARY BICYCLE

After 10 to 20 minutes of warm up exercises, follow this program daily:

First Two Weeks
1. Ride bicycle for 3 minutes
2. Do 10 Sit-ups
3. Ride for 3 minutes
4. Do 10 Push-ups
5. Ride for 3 minutes
6. Do 8 Side Leg Raises
7. Ride for 3 minutes
8. Do 8 Leg Sit-ups
9. Ride for 3 minutes

Third and Fourth Weeks
1. Ride bicycle for 4 minutes
2. Do 10 Sit-ups
3. Ride for 4 minutes
4. Do 10 Push-ups
5. Ride for 4 minutes
6. Do 10 Side Leg Raises
7. Ride for 4 minutes

Fifth and Sixth Weeks
1. Ride for 5 minutes
2. Do 12 Sit-ups
3. Ride for 5 minutes
4. Do 12 Push-ups
5. Ride for 5 minutes
6. Do 12 Leg Sit-ups
7. Ride for 5 minutes

Seventh and Eighth Weeks
1. Ride for 7 minutes
2. Do 20 Sit-ups
3. Ride for 7 minutes
4. Do 15 Push-ups
5. Ride for 7 minutes
6. Do 12 Leg Sit-ups
7. Ride for 7 minutes

Ninth and Tenth Weeks
1. Ride for 10 minutes
2. Do 20 Push-ups
3. Do 20 Sit-ups
4. Ride for 10 minutes
5. Do 15 Leg Sit-ups
6. Do 15 Side Leg Raises
7. Ride for 10 minutes

Eleventh and Twelfth Weeks
1. Ride for 15 minutes
2. Do 20 Sit-ups
3. Do 20 Push-ups
4. Do 20 Leg Raises
5. Ride for 15 minutes

Thirteenth and Fourteenth Weeks
1. Ride for 20 minutes
2. Do 25 Sit-ups
3. Do 25 Push-ups
4. Do 20 Leg Raises
5. Do 20 Side Leg Raises
6. Ride for 10 minutes

Fifteenth and Sixteenth Weeks
Ride bicycle for 25 to 30 minutes.

Now that you are conditioned and have developed a healthy cardio-vascular system, you can ride the bicycle 25 to 30 minutes per day non-stop. Make sure that before you ride the bicycle, you warm-up adequately and record your training pulse rate as specified.

WHY JOGGING ?

During the past fifteen years one of the most obvious changes in the American lifestyle has been a gradual increase in the number of people who exercise. A recent study indicated that forty-seven percent of people claim to exercise. This is double the number who made that claim sixteen years ago. The exercise boom is continually expanding. People now believe that exercise is helpful in promoting good health. If this is so, then which form of exercise is most helpful in promoting good health and in the prevention of heart disease?

It is true that all forms of physical activity bring about physiological benefits. Exercise generates a feeling of well-being and accomplishment. But in order to prevent heart disease, the exercise should have a primary purpose—to improve the cardiovascular system. An exercise that is rhythmic and increases pulse rate to 130 to 140 beats per minute and that lasts for 20 to 30 minutes is the answer. Jogging, swimming, stationary bicycle and jumping rope all stimulate the heart and increase the pulse rate and oxygen consumption of the cardiac muscle. By doing so, these exercises are rated very high in improving cardiovascular fitness and preventing heart disease. In golf, tennis, bowling, baseball or any other physical activity related to these types, the pulse rate is not kept high for a long enough period of time.

Today, jogging has developed into one of the most popular forms of exercise in this country, especially among more educated groups who place a higher value on personal health than anything else in life.

WHY IS JOGGING THE BEST EXERCISE ?

An analysis of jogging as a form of exercise indicates that there are two unique features of jogging.

Feature One

1. Jogging rates as the simplest and the most natural form of exercise
2. It requires no special skills
3. Requires no special equipment or clothing
4. Requires no special facilities such as gym or indoor track
5. Has no age or sex limitation.

Feature Two

1. Jogging reduces the resting pulse rate
2. Increases the strength of the cardiac muscle
3. Normalizes both the systolic and diastolic blood pressures
4. Increases metabolism of the body, helping to reduce weight
5. Produces new capillaries in the cardiac muscle and sets up collateral circulation
6. Reduces emotional tension by stimulating the parasympathetic nervous system
7. Increases the diameter of the major blood vessels consequently preventing hardening and plugging of the arteries.

CAN JOGGING BE DANGEROUS ?

As it was indicated earlier, jogging is the best and most suitable exercise for the heart, however it can also be a dangerous one for the cardiovascular system. Failure to understand your functional capacity and level of physical fitness can be dangerous as well as fatal. There is a tendency with beginning joggers to go all out and try to improve themselves the very first day. Such a practice is not beneficial to the heart and may leave a lasting scar on the heart muscle, leading to eventual heart disease. The beginning jogger must realize that their endurance may be low and their cardiovascular system not ready for hard and strenuous exercise. They need to take it easy, progressing gradually. They must bear in mind that improvement in cardiovascular fitness cannot be accomplished overnight. It takes time and effort.

The following program has been designed for those who wish to begin a jogging program:

First Two Weeks
1. Jog   2 minutes
2. Walk   2 minutes
3. Repeat 12 to 15 times

Second Two Weeks
1. Jog   4 minutes
2. Walk   2 minutes
3. Repeat 6 to 7 times

Third Two Weeks
1. Jog   6 minutes
2. Walk   3 minutes
3. Repeat 4 to 5 times

Fourth Two Weeks
1. Jog   10 minutes
2. Walk   5 minutes
3. Repeat 2 to 3 times

Fifth Two Weeks
1. Jog   15 minutes
2. Walk   5 minutes

Sixth Two Weeks
1. Jog   20 minutes

* NOTE:
After the sixth two week program, you can increase your jogging to 30 minutes. Now you are well trained. Your body is completely adjusted to the work out.

WEIGHT TRAINING

Today we need more muscular strength, endurance, flexibility and a stronger bone structure than ever before. We are a population no longer involved in activities that can develop strength and stamina. We are losing our muscle tone and endurance earlier in life, enabling our bodies to give in to the aging process early on so that a person age thirty does not have the strength and vitality to stand against the forces of aging. Our muscles, tendons and ligaments are so weak that they can easily become stressed or fractured. Inability to maintain good balance subjects us to falls and bone fractures.

Weight training develops strength, endurance and builds up strong bones, joints and ligaments. In weight training every single muscle is involved in exercise. It is the only exercise that provides an excellent blood supply to the facial muscles, whereas all other exercises reduce blood supply to the facial muscles. Because weight training increases blood supply to the facial muscles, it slows down the aging process of our skin and prevents early occurrence of facial wrinkles. That is why people who work out with weights look so much younger than people who participate in other forms of exercise.

Weight training also plays a very important role in the reduction of stress. By exerting maximum pressure against a weight, it releases emotional tension. Today it is recommended to all people over twenty-five years of age to engage in weight training activities, in order to improve and maintain their strength and endurance and to relieve emotional stress.

Weight Training Program

A weight training program should include six basic exercises.

1. **Curl.**

The purpose of this exercise is to develop the bicep muscles which are located in the front of the upper arms. Begin this exercise with a barbell at thigh level. Curl the barbell to chest level and return it to the starting position. Repeat 6 times.

2. **Squat.**

The purpose of this exercise is to develop hips and thigh muscles. Begin exercise with barbell across the back of the shoulders. Next, bend the knees while keeping the back straight. Return to starting position. Repeat 6 times.

3. **Military Press.**

Lift barbell to the chest and raise the weight directly overhead by keeping the elbows straight. Return weight back to chest. Repeat 6 times.

4. **Toe Raising.**

The purpose here is to develop calf muscles. Begin exercise with barbell across back of the shoulders. Rise up on the toes, keeping the body straight and the feet 12 inches apart. Return to the starting position. Repeat 6 times.

5. **Bench Press.**

The purpose is to develop pectoral muscles. Lie on a bench with feet flat on the floor and barbell resting on the chest. Press barbell straight up. Keep arms straight. Return barbell to starting position. Repeat 6 times.

6. Pull Up.

This exercise develops back muscles. Begin with barbell resting against the front of the thighs. Pull barbell straight up so that it is parallel to the shoulders. Return barbell to starting position. Repeat 6 times.

Rules You Should Follow

1. Know your strength capability. To find out, select a weight and lift it 6 times. If it is easy to lift, increase the weight. If it is difficult, reduce the weight.
2. Breathe in before lifting. Breathe out after the lift has been completed.
3. Rest 30 seconds between each lift in order that muscles can recover.
4. Warm up for 10 minutes prior to engaging in weight lifting activity to prevent injuries to your muscles and joints.
5. Make sure that your equipment and the place you are exercising is safe.
6. Do not exercise after eating. It is better to exercise with an empty stomach.

CARBOHYDRATE LOADING

The capacity of the liver and muscles to store glycogen can be increased almost 100 percent by manipulation of the diet in relation to athletic activities. This procedure is known as "carbohydrate loading". It is used by athletes to improve the endurance in prolonged activities, such as long distance running. This practice of dieting has become popular especially among marathon runners. The basis for such a dietary plan is that in short and moderate exercise, muscles use fatty acid for energy. But, during vigorous and prolonged activities such as marathons, muscles switch to glycogen as a source of energy. The basic idea behind carbohydrate loading is that an increase in the amount of glycogen stored in the muscles will enhance the athletes endurance. A normal level of glycogen in an athlete with a normal mixed diet is 1.5 grams of glycogen per 100 grams of muscle. However, if an athlete switches to a diet high in carbohydrate, the muscle glycogen will go up 2.5 grams per 100 grams of muscle. With carbohydrate loading, we can increase muscle glycogen to 5 grams per 100 grams of muscle.

The procedure of carbohydrate loading is as follows:

1. An athlete must exercise vigorously 4 to 6 days prior to a contest, consuming a low carbohydrate diet. This effort exhausts the stored glycogen in the muscles.
2. On the day before the competition, athletes switch to a high carbohydrate diet, with light exercise.

It has been shown that the endurance of a well trained athlete is much less apt to be impaired by carbohydrate loading, than that of a less trained athlete. In trained athletes, utilization of glycogen is at a much lower rate than that of an untrained person. This is due to an athlete's ability to utilize glycogen more efficiently.

CHAPTER 7

WHERE DO WE GET OUR NUTRITION KNOWLEDGE

Today in America, newspapers, television talk shows and magazine articles are the principle sources of nutrition information for the general public. These sources have a strong influence on food trends and nutrition beliefs for millions of consumers. According to recent studies, the majority of the available information does not have any scientific basis and is not reliable data. Media sources promote pills, herbs and drugs for losing weight and curing a variety of diseases.

Nutritional hustlers are cleaning up financially by stalking our fears and hopes with misleading information and credentials. They dominate television info-mercials and commercial publications. Television talk show hosts love them because they attract large audiences. These hustlers advise people that if you eat poorly, do not worry, just take my food supplement. They claim that natural vitamins are better than synthetic vitamins, that brown eggs are better than white eggs and that brown sugar is better than white sugar so that they can sell these products at much higher prices. In actuality, there is no difference between these products. White eggs are just as good as brown eggs. Synthetic vitamins have the same effect as natural vitamins. Another group of quacks claim they can identify a person's nutritional deficiencies by hair analysis. In fact, hair analysis after being studied, has been found to be useless as a screening device to detect nutritional deficiency.

Television talk show hosts give a boost to the diet industry quacks when they ask what all these herbs do for you. They quickly reply that their products can improve vigor, vitality and memory, as well as fight against insomnia and cancer. Other quacks buy 30 minutes of television time to promote the power of enzymes. They claim that their enzyme products taken by mouth aid digestion and prevent acid reflux, constipation and bloatedness. But in actuality, enzymes taken by mouth do not function as enzymes within the body. These quacks also tell us all the wonderful things our bodies can experience by taking their vitamins, minerals, herbs and enzymes and that harmful things happen to our bodies if we neglect to heed their advice. They conveniently neglect to inform listeners that a well balanced diet can provide all the nutrients that your body needs. Health food quacks promote many numbers of unreliable supplements with all kinds of claims. Their claims are based upon faulty explanations of animal research. The most notorious of such product claims was tryptophan, an amino acid. For a long time it was marketed as a product for insomnia, depression and weight loss. Then in 1989, the use of this product caused a serious health hazzard called eosinophelia mylgio syndrome, a rare disease characterized by swelling arms and legs, skin rash, fever and joint pain. The most widespread area of false information today is in the promotion of health foods and health food supplements. A large number of people are being misled concerning the need for these products. Health food industries use the vast and growing folklore surrounding nutrition which is being built up by pseudoscientific literature in books, pamphlets and magazines. As a result, millions of people are attempting self-medication for both imaginary and real illnesses with a multitude of more or less irrational food items. Health food quackery today can only be compared to the patent medicine craze which reached its highest peak in the last century.

Present day nutrition scientists agree that most chronic diseases such as heart disease, cancer, diabetes and digestive diseases are all rooted in the food we eat. Our diet can determine how we feel, look and act. The food we eat can physiologically and psychologically affect our mood, our thinking, our energy, our self-confidence and our power of determination. In short, food can influence your zest for life and the fulfillment you get from life. Physiologically food affects our vigor, energy and vitality as well as our level of fatigue and exhaustion.

Food has the ability to determine how we feel, look and act. It can influence whether you are grouchy or cheerful, whether you think clearly or confused, get pleasure from your work or make it a drudgery. Our diet can also make the difference between a day ending with freshness, leading to a delightful evening or with fatigue, forcing us early to bed.

Most people talking about nutrition are food faddists or celebrities who have no scientific training. They peddle a tremendous amount of misinformation . The most important fact regarding good nutrition concerns not how much we eat, but what we eat. Today foods are high in fat, salt and chemical additives, which are responsible for most of the health problems we face, especially the problem of obesity. If we reduce the amount of fat, salt and chemical additives in our diets and add a little physical activity to our daily lives, we will be able to combat most of the major health problems, including obesity, as it was done by generations before us. Based upon the misleading and often confusing information regarding nutrition and its effect on health, I have devoted a portion of this book to educate the public on basic nutrition.

Carbohydrates

Carbohydrate is the ideal energy source for most body functions. No food substances can provide a better fuel to the brain and nervous system than carbohydrates. The central nervous system is entirely dependent on carbohydrates. Other food substances, such as protein, fat and alcohol are not efficient fuels. If they are used in larger amounts they may produce very harmful effects. For example, a larger amount of protein in the body increases uric acid and causes kidney problems. Large usage of fat is responsible for heart disease and hardening of the blood vessels.

Carbohydrates have always been an important source of energy for people around the world. Lack of carbohydrate in the diet has been identified with causing tension, mental confusion and poor reaction. A person whose blood sugar falls below normal becomes progressively more irritable, grouchy, moody, depressed and uncooperative. Since the brain can derive its energy only from carbohydrate foods, danger of blackout or fainting can occur if the supply falls below normal levels. On the other hand, if a diet provides adequate amounts of carbohydrates, blood sugar goes up and energy is easily produced, resulting in feeling better, feeling full of drive and the ability to think quickly and clearly. Your attitude is gracious and cheerful. Your disposition is at its best.

Classification of Carbohydrates in Terms of Health

Carbohydrates are divided into two groups.
1. Complex Carbohydrates
2. Non-Complex Carbohydrates
This classification system is based on their effects on health.

Complex Carbohydrates:

Complex carbohydrates occur in natural forms not altered by industrial process. They are fruits, vegetables, rice, potatoes to name a few. These carbohydrate foods have special characteristics:

A. They are very high in vitamins, minerals, fiber, natural sugar and natural water.

B. They are very low in salt, cholesterol, calories and chemical additives.

Non-Complex Carbohydrates:

These foods are altered through industrial processing. They are:
A. Low in vitamins, minerals and fiber.
B. High in fat, additives, salt and calories

COMPLEX CARBOHYDRATE

Complex carbohydrate foods such as corn, rice, potato, wheat bread, natural fruits and vegetables can provide good fuel to the body and maintain the blood sugar within the normal range. These foods prevent blood sugar fluctuation, which is very important in the prevention of fatigue. Fruits and vegetables provide vitamins, minerals and good sources of fiber to the body. On the other hand, concentrated sugars and products made from them such as pastries, cakes and soft drinks are absorbed rapidly into the blood circulation in a matter of minutes and raise the blood sugar very high. This rapid rise in blood sugar over-stimulates the healthy pancreas to pour insulin into the blood. The insulin in turn, causes the liver and muscles to withdraw sugar and store it as fat, thus preventing it from being lost in the urine. As the consumption of concentrated sugar continues, more sugar will pour into the blood, calling for the pancreas to send more insulin and the pancreas obeys. The blood sugar drops below normal as a result of too much insulin. Then, a person begins to experience the symptoms of hypoglycemia which can be fatigue, anxiety, stress, headache, sweating and/or dizziness. If the consumption of concentrated sugar products continues, the pancreas becomes fatigued and weakens. It no longer will produce an adequate amount of insulin to keep the blood sugar in the normal range. The blood sugar goes up and it cannot be controlled without medication. This is the beginning stage of diabetes.

Digestion of Carbohydrates

Before carbohydrates can produce energy, they must be converted into sufficiently small units to pass through the walls of the intestine into the bloodstream. The process by which complex carbohydrates such as pasta or rice are reduced to their component units is one aspect of digestion. Virtually all the changes involved are brought about by an enzyme called amylase. Amylase is present in two digestive juices:

A) The saliva in the mouth

B) The pancreatic juice in the small intestine

The salivary amylase mixes with the food in the mouth and converts it to simpler carbohydrates called dextrins. No digestion of carbohydrates takes place in the stomach because the stomach possesses no starch splitting enzyme. From the stomach, the digestive mass passes to the small intestine where pancreatic amylase attack complex carbohydrates and convert them into glucose and fructose making them ready for absorption into the blood stream. From the intestinal wall, the simple sugars are carried to the liver. In the liver, part of glucose is converted into glycogen and stored in the liver and part of it is released into the bloodstream to be carried to various cells in the body. Most glucose will be utilized as an immediate source of energy for the cells. The nerve and lung cells depend entirely on glucose as a source of energy. The excessive sugar in the liver is converted into fat and then transported in the bloodstream to the adipose tissue cells.

Characteristics of Non-Complex Carbohydrates:

A) These carbohydrates such as sugar, cake and pastry are very high in salt, cholesterol, fat, calories, chemical additives and sugar.

B) They are very low in vitamins, minerals and fiber. Examples of non-complex carbohydrates are cake, pie, potato chips, cookies and muffins.

These foods are the underlying source for many human illnesses such as diabetes, constipation and digestive disorders.

Classification of Carbohydrates

In terms of chemical structure, carbohydrates are divided into three groups.
1. Mono-Saccharides
2. Di-Saccharides
3. Poly-Saccharides

Mono-Saccharides:

These carbohydrates are made up from three groups.
1. Glucose
2. Fructose
3. Galactose
Glucose is found in fruits, vegetables, honey and in the human blood.
Fructose is formed together with glucose in fruits. The sweetness of the fruit is due to the amount of fructose it contains. The higher the fructose, the sweeter the fruit.
Galactose is found only in mothers milk. It is essential for infant nutrition.

Di-Saccharides:

These carbohydrates are made up from two simple sugars.
These are divided into three groups:
1. Lactose
2. Sucrose
3. Maltose
Lactose is found only in milk. The human milk has more lactose than cows milk. Lactose is made up from glucose and galactose and it is not very sweet.

Lactose Intolerance

Some people cannot digest milk. They lack an enzyme. In such circumstances, lactose passes into the large intestine where it is fermented by the intestinal bacteria, causing diarrhea, gas and abdominal pain. Those whose ancestors come from the areas around Italy, Greece and North Africa tend to have a problem digesting milk. Italian, Spanish, Greek, Jewish and Black people are included in this group. The reason being that these nationalities consumed cheese rather than milk, therefore they did not develop the digestive enzyme for milk, called "amylase". These people will not have tolerance for milk. For those who cannot tolerate milk, cheese should be used as a source of calcium. Cheese does not contain lactose. During the cheese making process lactose is converted into lactic acid, which does not require amylase.

Sucrose

Sucrose is found in sugar cane, sugar beets, maple syrup and fruits. Table sugar is made up from sucrose.

Poly-Saccharides

Poly-Saccharides are composed of glucose linked together to form very large molecules. Poly-Saccharides are divided into three groups called Starches, Cellulose, and Glycogen.

Starches occur in plant seeds such as potatoes, wheat, rice, corn, and oats. Starches represent half the dietary carbohydrates. Each plant develops a starch characteristic of its species. The starch of potato can be distinguished from that of rice. Animals store a limited amount of carbohydrates. It is stored primarily in the liver and muscles. An adult human stores only about 340 grams of glycogen in the body. The capacity of the liver and muscles to store glycogen can be increased by manipulating the diet in association with exercise. This procedure is known as carbohydrate loading.

Cellulose is widely distributed among plants and is the only component of dietary fiber having a fibrous structure. The basic unit of cellulose is glucose. Cellulose cannot be utilized by humans as a source of energy because humans do not have any enzyme to digest cellulose. Animals such as cows and horses can utilize it for energy but cellulose has a tremendous beneficial effect on human health. It protects the digestive system from cancer, constipation and many other digestive problems which are mentioned in the section devoted to The Effects of Fiber in Human Nutrition.

Glycogen. Foods have very little glycogen. Glycogen has been called animal starch and is manufactured in the liver and muscles from glucose. Glycogen serves as a source of stored energy which the liver can easily break down into glucose when needed to maintain the blood sugar level or to use for energy. Most of the glycogen is stored in the muscles and in the liver. Glycogen plays a very important role in physical exercise and carbohydrate loading.

FOODS HIGH IN FIBER

Complex Carbohydrates

GROUP A BREADS (Whole Wheat)

Rye Bread
Corn
Pasta
Potato
Rice

GROUP B FRUITS

Apple
Cantaloupe
Citrus Fruits
Grapes
Grapefruit
Honeydew
Pineapple
Pear
Plum
Watermelon
Peaches
Prunes
Dried Fruits

GROUP C VEGETABLES

Asparagus
Broccoli
Brussel Sprouts
Carrots
Cabbage
Cauliflower
Celery
Corn
Eggplant
Endive
Lettuce
Green Beans
Lima Beans
All other beans
Mushrooms

Okra
Peas (all types)
Radishes
Spinach
Squash
Sauerkraut
Tomatoes
Turnips
Watercress

GROUP D CEREALS

Oatmeal
Shredded Wheat
Bran Cereal
Puffed Rice
Raw, unprocessed bran

GROUP E BREADS

Whole Wheat
Cracked Wheat
Buck Wheat
Corn Bread

NOTE:
You can have any other vegetable or fruit that is not listed in this group provided they are not altered.

FOODS LOW IN FIBER

GROUP A

White Rice
Cream of Wheat
Farina
White Bread
Pasta
Pastries
Pie
Cakes
Macaroni
Spaghetti
Noodles

FOODS WITHOUT FIBER

GROUP B

Beef
Veal
Lamb
Fish
Shrimp
Lobster
Ham
Turkey
Tuna
Pork

Eggs
Margarine
Vegetable Oils
Ketchup
Chicken
Bacon
Butter
Cream
Salad Dressing
Corn Oil
Olive Oil
Ice Cream

CHAPTER 8

FATS

Fats are a part of every meal and are familiar to everyone, such as butter, vegetables oils, lard and margarine being common examples. The average American consumes about one-forth of a pound of fat (110 grams) per day, a practice not within its nutritional hazards. In Japan or China a very small percent (6%) of the diet comes from fat; whereas Americans consume more than forty percent fat in their total calorie intake. Fat is an organic substance insoluble in water, but soluble in alcohol. The principle foods contributing fat to the diet are not only butter, margarine, lard and vegetable oils, but invisible fats found in cream, milk products, egg yolk, avocados and nuts.

Classification of Fats:

Fats are divided into two groups:
1. Saturated Fats
2. Unsaturated Fats

Saturated Fats:

This kind of fat comes from animal origins. They are solid at room temperature. Fats found in meat, butter, chicken and dairy products are saturated. These fats are major contributors to cardiovascular disease, cancer, high blood pressure, high cholesterol and obesity.

Unsaturated Fats:
These fats come from plants, such as corn, olives, nuts and vegetables and are in a liquid state. They are not harmful to the individual health, but excessive use of this fat will contribute to obesity. Each gram of fat produces nine calories no matter what its origin (animal or plant).

Functions of Fats:
Fats play a very important role in the human body. Without fat the body cannot carry on its vital functions.
These functions are:
1. Production of energy
2. Protection of the vital organs
3. Production of hormones
4. Insulation of the body
5. Protection of the skin from radiation
6. Absorption of Vitamins A, D, E and K

DIGESTION OF FATS

Fats are digested primarily in the small intestine. No digestion of fat takes place in the stomach. The function of the stomach in relation to fat digestion is to liquidize it. As fat enters the small intestine, the presence of fat stimulates the intestinal wall to secrete a hormone that is carried to the gall bladder by the blood. This hormone stimulates the contraction of the gall bladder, thereby forcing bile into the common duct and then into the small intestine.
Bile has several important functions:
1. It stimulates peristalsis, which is a natural movement of the digestive tract to help move the bowel.
2. To neutralize acid environment so as to provide the optimum condition for the digestion of fat.
3. To increase the effectiveness of enzyme action on fat digestion.

Fatty food reduces the mobility of the digestive tract. Foods high in fat remain in the stomach longer than those that are low in fat. Fried foods are digested at a much slower rate. Lack of bile acid interferes with digestion of fat causing gas, bloatedness and constipation.

Lack of bile acid is caused by:

1. Gallstone blocking the common bile duct
2. Infection of the common bile duct

METABOLISM OF FATS:

Fat enters the cells and it is used in several ways:

1. Some of the fats are oxidized and produce energy
2. Others are stored in the cells
3. Some others are used for the synthesis of hormones
4. The remaining fat is stored in the adipose tissues and forms a layer known as subcutaneous fat

CONSUMPTION OF FAT IN AMERICA

The predominant nutrient in the American diet is fat. Some of these dietary fats are identified as visible fats and oils such as butter, margarine, solid fat and fat surrounding meat. The other fats are called invisible fats including that fat marbled throughout meat fibers, in eggs, in milk, nuts and legumes. Today, sixty percent of the dietary fat comes from animal sources and forty percent from vegetable sources. In 1910, fat consumption was approximately 125 grams per day, but by 1980, the consumption of fat increased to 168 grams per day. The consumption of fat in the American diet is much higher than other countries in the world. For instance, consumption of fat in Europe is 109 grams per day.

There is a very strong correlation between fat consumption and cardiovascular disease. As the consumption of fat increases, the instance of cardiovascular diseases, cancer and obesity increases. To prevent disease and improve our health and well-being, we must take the following into consideration:

1. A reduction in the total fat calories from 45% to 25%
2. A reduction of total fat from animal sources
3. Remove visible fat from meat and poultry
4. Use more fat from vegetable sources
5. Increase the consumption of complex carbohydrates
6. Avoid the consumption of fried foods.

WHY SHOULD WE REDUCE OUR SATURATED FAT INTAKE ?

Saturated fats in the diet will affect the level of serum cholesterol by changing the number of receptors to a low density cholesterol in the liver. When saturated fats are decreased in the diet, the number of high density cholesterol receptors are increased in the liver. The liver is the major organ in the body for pulling and clearing low density cholesterol from the bloodstream and sending it to the digestive system for excretion. Therefore our goal should be to reduce our total saturated fat consumption to not more than ten percent of total calorie intake.

TIPS TO REDUCE SATURATED FATS IN YOUR DIET

To reduce the amount of saturated fats in the diet, we must do the following:

1. Steam, bake or broil foods
2. Use seasonings to improve the taste, such as lemon, garlic, onion and other non-salt spices
3. Use corn and olive oils in place of animal fats
4. Replace whole milk with skim or one percent milk
5. Use plain, low-fat yogurt in place of sour cream
6. Trim all visible fat from meat and poultry
7. Remove all skin from poultry before cooking

8. Use a non-stick pan for cooking so that there is no need to use fat
9. Avoid high fat cheese
10. Avoid using coconut oil, palm oil, butter, margarine, coffee creamer, ice cream, cream cheese, sausage and fried foods

CHOLESTEROL

Cholesterol occurs only in foods of animal origin. Liver, kidney and eggs contain the largest amount of cholesterol among foods. Other sources of cholesterol in the diet are meats, shell fish and dairy products. Cholesterol is a form of fat. The body can produce all that it needs and therefore is not dependent on dietary cholesterol.

Cholesterol plays many important roles in the body:

1. It is a very important structural component of all cells in the body
2. It is essential for normal development of the brain and nervous system
3. Cholesterol is the important substance in the skin that makes it impervious to water
4. The breakdown of cholesterol by the liver produces bile acid, without which digestion of fat cannot occur
5. Cholesterol is a vital component of many hormones, including sex hormones
6. Cholesterol in the skin, with help from the sun, produces Vitamin D. Vitamin D is essential for absorption of calcium in the digestive system
7. Cholesterol also protects skin against radiation (skin cancer)

DANGER OF HIGH CHOLESTEROL

Blood cholesterol comes from two sources. Most of the bodies cholesterol is synthesized by the liver, but some is obtained through the diet. Cholesterol has repeatedly shown to be associated with a high risk of coronary artery disease and myocardial infarction. Further research has drawn a distinction between high density lipoprotein (HDL) and low density lipoprotein (LDL). Now it is believed that the balance between HDL and LDL is more important than total cholesterol in the blood. The risk of coronary heart disease increases as LDL increases and HDL decreases. That is because HDL promotes the removal of excess cholesterol from the cells and its excretion from the body. In contrast, LDL picks up the cholesterol from ingested fats and from cells that synthesize it in the body and delivers it to the blood vessels. The concentration of cholesterol in the cells within the lining of the arteries contributes to the build up of arteriosclerotic plaques. All experts agree that we must keep our blood cholesterol in the normal range. No one should have a cholesterol above 200, especially those who are overweight and those who have a family history of heart disease. The ratio of HDL and LDL must be kept low. You must keep the high density cholesterol above 50 mg and your low density cholesterol under 130 mg. Low density blood cholesterol is the major cause of heart disease. It is vitally important that we should lower the LDL cholesterol. Numerous studies suggested that several factors play a vital role in the reduction of LDL. Among them are:

1. Decrease dietary cholesterol
2. Decrease calories from saturated fat
3. Decrease calories from fat
4. Increase fiber in your diet (fruits, vegetables, whole grain products)
5. Reduce body weight
6. Participate in aerobic exercise

Dietary fat is also associated with the second leading cause of death in the United States, which is cancer. A diet high in fat is a major factor in the development of breast, colon, rectal and prostrate cancers. Four major diseases are also associated with high intake of animal fat and a high percentage of other body fat. These diseases are:

1. Obesity
2. Cardiovascular disease
3. Diabetes
4. Cancer

CARDIOVASCULAR DISEASE

Cardiovascular disease is a disorder of the heart and blood vessels. These diseases include heart attack, stroke, high blood pressure and atherosclerosis. These diseases are responsible for one out of every two deaths in America.

The major risk factors are:

A) High blood cholesterol

B) Consumption of high dietary animal fats

HOW TO INCREASE HIGH DENSITY CHOLESTEROL

1. Increase the consumption of fish, especially blue fish and salmon
2. Increase fruits and vegetables in the diet
3. Increase whole grain products
4. Increase the level of physical activities
5. Avoid: Consumption of beef, pork and lamb
    Whole milk dairy products, such as cheese, butter and margarine
    Salad dressing and canned sauces

ESSENTIAL FATTY ACID

One of the most important reasons to include fat in the diet is to supply linoleic acid. Linoleic acid is an essential fatty acid and must be obtained from foods because the body is unable to synthesize it. Lack of this substance will produce certain symptoms.

Among them are:

1. Dry skin
2. Dermatitis
3. Damage to the hair follicle
4. Growth retardation

Sources of Linoleic Acid:

1. Corn oil
2. Sunflower oil
3. Soybean oil

To obtain a sufficient amount of linoleic acid, corn oil should be used for cooking. That is the reason I have included corn oil in my recipes. Fat is a very important substance and it has many vital functions in the body. Lack of fat in the diet causes many abnormalities. More vitally important is the type of fat in the diet. Some fat is used as part of the structure of every cell. The brain, nerves and skin need certain types of fats called essential fatty acids. Hormones and sex glands are made up of essential fatty acids which are linoleic acid, linolenic acid and arachidonic acid. Lack of these acids in the diet cause the hair to become dry and thin and the skin to become thick and scaly, especially the skin on the face. Excema also develops. By adding these essential fatty acids to the diet, the skin clears up and excema disappears.

A certain amount of fat is used in the body to stimulate the production of bile acid, which is essential for the digestion of fat. Low levels of bile acid causes abnormal digestion of fat, producing stomach gas, bloatedness and constipation. Abnormal fat digestion also prevents absorption of Vitamins A, D and K. Sources of essential fatty acids are corn oil, vegetable oil, soybean and cottonseed oil. Very little essential fatty acids are found in animal fats.

CHAPTER 9

PROTEINS

Proteins are the key components of all living organisms. Protein gets it name from a Greek word meaning "of first importance". They are essential constituents of blood and the nucleus of every cell. Twenty percent of body weight is composed of protein. Without protein, life cannot be sustained.

STRUCTURE OF PROTEIN

Protein is made up from carbon, oxygen, hydrogen and nitrogen. The basic units of protein are amino acids. When protein is digested in the body, it becomes an amino acid and it is the amino acid that enters the blood stream. There are 22 amino acids that the body needs to perform its major functions. Eight of these amino acids are essential and must be provided from the outside because the body cannot make them.

CLASSIFICATION OF PROTEIN

From a nutritional point of view, proteins are divided into two groups. They are:
1. Essential proteins
2. Nonessential proteins

Essential Proteins:

This type of protein comes from animal sources such as sea foods, beef, lamb, pork, eggs and dairy products. Without essential protein, growth and the maintenance of the body will be impaired and the body will not have the capacity to fight infections. The adult body needs 80 to 100 grams of essential protein per day. Pregnant women, children and people who are under emotional stress need more protein.

Sources of Essential Proteins:

All essential proteins come from animal sources. No essential proteins can be found in plant foods. Good sources of protein are:

Chicken	Turkey	Dairy Products
Eggs	Meat (lamb, pork, beef)	Fish (all types)
Shell fish		

Nonessential Proteins:

These types of proteins come from plant sources, such as corn, bread, rice, fruits, legumes and potatoes. Protein from plants cannot provide adequate amounts of essential protein to meet the requirements for growth and maintenance of the body. These proteins must be supplemented by animal protein. Combinations of essential protein and nonessential protein will provide all the nutrients that the body needs for growth and development of muscle tissue as well as for bone, blood and antibodies.

Sources of Nonessential Proteins:

Wheat	Corn	Rice
Pasta	Potato	Beans
Fruits	Vegetables	

To maintain our bodies in good health we need a high quality protein. Meat, fish, fowl, milk, cheese, yogurt and eggs are superior sources of high quality proteins. Proteins are made up from amino acids containing nitrogen, which are lacking in other food sources. Not only does the protein of milk differ from those of cereal, but the protein in all parts of our body varies due to the different combinations of amino acids which form them. When these proteins are eaten, the digestive process of a healthy person breaks them down into amino acids which pass into the blood and are then carried throughout the body. The cells select the amino acids they need, using them to construct new body tissue and for such vital substances as antibodies, hormones, enzymes and blood cells. Every second our body's protein is being broken down by enzymes in our cells, and if our health is to be maintained, then amino acids must be available for immediate replacement.

When our diet has more protein available than our body needs, the liver withdraws amino acids from the blood and changes them into storage proteins. These excessive proteins will be converted into glucose and fat by the liver, and the nitrogen of the protein will be excreted in the urine. The glucose and fat will be used for energy or will be stored as fat. Some of these essential amino acids are used for treatment of diseases.

The eight essential amino acids are:

Methionine	Phenylalanine	Threonine	Valine
Leucine	Isoleucine	Tryptophan	Lysine

Two other amino acids are essential for growth. During childhood the diet must supply them.

They are histidine and arginine. The value of any protein depends on the number and amount of essential amino acids it contains. Proteins containing the eight essential amino acids in generous amounts are called complete. If enough of any complete protein such as milk is taken, it alone can support health. A protein lacking one or more essential amino acid or supplying too little of an essential amino acid to support life is an incomplete protein. Protein from meat, fish, eggs, milk, steak, cheese and other animal sources have higher values for health than protein from vegetables, cereals, breads, potato and pasta.

Extensive research has been done with both animals and humans to find the specific symptoms of ill health that occur when certain amino acids are lacking. For example, when the diet of animals or babies lack tryptophan, methionine or isoleucine, the liver cannot produce the blood proteins albumin and globulin (antibodies), therefore urine can no longer be collected normally. Swelling known as edema and susceptibility to infection results. Methionine has been found to be particularly deficient in the diet of children with chronic rheumatic fever and of women suffering from the toxemia of pregnancy. In animals, a lack of tryptophan or methionine causes the hair to fall out. Lack of phenylalanine causes the eyes to become blood shot or cataracts to form.

Functions of Proteins:

Proteins provide a key life force. They are crucial to the minute by minute regulation and maintenance of the various functions of our bodies. Vital body functions such as blood clotting, fluid balance, hormone and enzyme production and cell repair all require protein. Our bodies are largely made up from protein, including skin, hair, nails, bones, muscles, brain and all internal organs. Only when high quality protein is supplied can each cell act normally and keep itself in constant repair. When we receive an inadequate amount of good quality protein, cells lose their elasticity, strength and energy.

Protein Builds and Repairs Tissues:

Lack of protein causes the cells, tissues, muscles and bones to become weak. The heart cannot push the blood through the blood vessels and the lungs cannot bring in fresh air, causing the blood pressure to go up. Because of this, less nutrients can be delivered to the tissues, resulting in fatigue, lack of energy and emotional stress. Another cause of fatigue, which is common, is anemia or lack of red blood cells which are made up almost entirely from protein. Red blood cells carry oxygen to the cells where the oxygen combines with food to produce energy. Low levels of red cells in the blood circulation is an indication of anemia or lack of energy.

Protein Prevents Infection:

Adequate protein is needed to produce various white blood cells. These white cells in the blood help to protect the body from invasion of bacterias. They are the armed forces of the body that guard us twenty-four hours a day. Some of these cells circulate in the blood and in the lymph system. Others are stationed in the walls of blood vessels, in the air sacs of the lungs, and in other tissues. When bacteria invades the body, these cells attack and destroy them right away. When the number of these cells decline, the body loses it's immunity and becomes infected.

Protein Maintains Water Balance:

Protein in the blood is responsible for maintaining the water level in the body. Pressure inside arteries pushes the blood into the capillaries and then into the tissues in order to supply nutrients to these tissues. The pressure produced by protein in the blood attracts the fluid back into the blood stream, thus controlling fluid balance in the circulation. Whenever the level of protein supply becomes inadequate, edema results. Edema leads to many serious medical problems, among them are heart damage, high blood pressure, respiratory problems and joint pain. It also causes fatigue, anxiety and lack of sleep.

Proteins Build Enzymes:

All our energy in the body is produced by enzymes. Enzymes are organic substances whose principle component is protein. Enzymes are necessary for digestion of foods in the digestive system. Enzymes break down foods into small particles which can be dissolved in water and passed into the circulation. The stomach, small intestine and pancreas can only produce enzymes when the supply of protein is adequate. The stomach walls, as well as the intestine and colon walls, must be kept strong in order to have a good digestive process.

How to Select Good Protein:

As it was discussed previously, protein plays a very important role in growth and maintenance of the body. However, the type of protein in the diet is one factor we must be concerned with. Protein from certain sources contain not only saturated fat, but growth hormones which are responsible for various cancers in man. The protein of lamb, beef and pork contain a lot of saturated fats and growth hormones. Proteins from these animal sources should be reduced in the diet as much as possible.

Problems associated with these animals are:

1. They store fat not only in between the muscle and skin, but also inside the muscle itself. That is the reason no matter what you do, you still will get a lot of saturated fat from these sources.

2. Growth hormones are injected into these animals for two reasons—To increase body mass and so that farmers can shorten the length of maturation of these animals. It is a very profitable method for cattle ranchers and dangerous for consumers.

In order to obtain good protein, we must consume our protein from the following sources:

Chicken	Turkey	Sea foods
Legume	Whole grains	Low fat dairy products

Who Should Increase Protein Intake:

There are special groups of people who must consume more protein in their diets.

They are:
1. Pregnant women who must support the growth of the fetus
2. People who had surgery
3. People who are under stress
4. People engaged in vigorous physical activities
5. Children in the process of growth

DIGESTION OF PROTEIN

Inside the mouth, nothing happens to protein except that it is crushed and mixed with saliva. When protein reaches the stomach, it faces a very strong acid. There, the acid helps to denature or split the protein so that the stomach enzymes can attack it and break it down into small pieces. Even though the stomach walls are made up from protein, the stomach acid and enzymes do not attack them because they are the only proteins in the body designed to resist strong acid. The stomach wall is protected by a coat of mucus, secreted by the stomach cells. By the time the denatured protein arrives to the intestine, it is broken down into smaller pieces. In the small intestine the acid delivered by the stomach is neutralized by alkaline juice from the pancreas, making it possible for intestinal enzymes to accomplish the final breakdown of the protein. Digestion continues until almost all proteins are broken down into amino acids.

Absorption of Protein:

Absorption of protein takes place all along the small intestine. The cells of the small intestine capture the amino acids and then release them into the bloodstream. Once they are circulating in the bloodstream, the amino acids are available to be taken up by any cell in the body. The cells can then make protein, either for their own use or for secretion into the lymph or blood systems for other uses such as enzymes, hormones or antibodies. The breakdown of protein foods in the stomach is accomplished by pepsin and in the small intestine it is carried out by tripsin.

The Best Way to Obtain Proper Protein:

For optimal growth and well being, the human body requires a combination of essential (animal) and nonessential (plant) protein. We cannot carry on the vital physiological activities of life without animal protein. Therefore a daily diet must contain some animal products, perhaps at about four ounces of animal protein per day. The rest may come from plant protein. When we combine animal protein with plant protein in the diet, both proteins become essential protein. A good example of this food combination is:

1. Cheese sandwich
2. Turkey sandwich
3. Chicken with rice
4. Beef with potatoes
5. Salad with turkey
6. Salad with cheese
7. Pasta with cheese
8. Sea food with rice
9. Tuna sandwich
10. Varieties of legumes with chicken, fish, turkey, beef, dairy products
11. Yogurt with fruit
12. Chicken soup
13. Egg sandwich
14. Cereal with milk

Such diets will promote both growth and maintenance of the body not only during growth periods, but also during adult life. It should be stressed that consuming large amounts of animal protein not only increases your risk of cardiovascular disease, but it also elevates the level of uric acid in the blood. A higher uric acid in the blood is responsible for gout. In addition, a higher uric acid level disturbs the normal range of pH of the blood. When the pH level of blood is disturbed it will effect all physiological functions of the vital organs.

VEGETARIANS

For many countries over the world, a vegetarian diet is used as an alternative diet by a large number of people. But since 1970, especially in the Western world, many young people most of whom come from middle and upper middle class backgrounds turned to vegetarian foods for a variety of reasons:

1. For some people it represents a form of religion or spiritual release through which they hope to purify their bodies and find a place in heaven or an "eternal world".

2. For another group, the vegetarian diet represents a form of rejection of many aspects of affluent society.

3. The vegetarian diet serves as a healer for other people. They believe that foods can replace medicine. They use vegetarian foods to heal diseases and illness.

4. Still there are people who use a vegetarian diet to slow down the aging process and eventually find the fountain of youth.

Vegetarians are divided into four groups:

1. **True Vegetarian.** This group believes that all life is sacred, and that no life should be destroyed. They do not consume any animal products or by products. These are religious groups living in India. True vegetarians are likely to suffer serious nutritional problems such as:

A) Vitamin deficiencies of Vitamins A, E, D, K and Vitamin B12

B) Mineral deficiencies of Iron, Calcium, Potassium and Zinc

C) Lack of energy. Energy supplied by vegetarian foods is not sufficient to provide an ample amount of energy to perform physical activities

2. **Lacto-Vegetarian.** This group consumes all vegetable foods plus dairy products such as yogurt, cheese, milk and butter. They avoid animal foods such as meat, poultry, sea food and eggs.

3. **Ovo-Lacto Vegetarian.** This group avoids all animal products except eggs and dairy products. They consume, eggs, cheese, butter, yogurt, milk and buttermilk, plus all vegetarian foods such as fruits, vegetables, legumes and whole grain products.

4. **Quasi-Vegetarian.** This group avoids all animal products except fish and sea foods. They do not consume eggs or dairy products.

CHAPTER 10

VITAMINS

The history of vitamins, their discovery and effects on the deficiency diseases is very fascinating. Vitamin investigation began with the search for unknown accessory dietary factors that would prevent or cure the classic deficiency diseases such as scurvy, rickets, pellagra, night blindness and hemorrhagic disease of newborns, to name a few. Through these elucidations of the etiologic role of vitamins, deficiencies in those diseases are among the brightest chapters in nutritional history. Although history cites evidence that the benefits of vitamins date as far back as the ancient Egyptians, scientific knowledge of vitamins dates back only to the close of the nineteenth century.

Christian Elgkman, in 1897, described a disease in chickens resembling beriberi in man. He induced this disease by feeding milled rice to chickens. The symptoms could be cured by feeding rice polishings. This recognition of the importance of other factors besides carbohydrates, fats and proteins in promoting health stimulated investigations by other workers which led to the modern concept of vitamins. Research in the field of vitamins was promoted by young biologist, Dr. Casimer Funk, who in 1912, at the age of 28, used the word "vitamin" meaning essential. In 1914, he wrote the first book on vitamins. He proposed that the dietary deficiency diseases of beriberi, scurvy, pellagra and rickets were caused by a lack in the diet of special substances which we call vitamins. By 1920, it was suggested that vitamins should be classified into fat and water soluble vitamins and it was accepted by the scientific community.

WHAT IS A VITAMIN ?

A vitamin is an organic compound other than protein, fat or carbohydrate. Vitamins are essential for growth, production of energy and maintenance of good health. Animals fed on pure fat, protein, carbohydrate, water and minerals failed to grow because they lacked vitamins. Most foods contain a good supply of vitamins, but today foods are processed and do not contain adequate amounts of vitamins, therefore most people lack vitamins.

CHARACTERISTICS OF VITAMINS:

1. Vitamins are not food, therefore they cannot satisfy hunger
2. The human body cannot produce vitamins. They must come from outside sources.
3. Each vitamin has a specific function in the body.
4. Some vitamins are fat soluble and others are water soluble, therefore they must be taken with food.
5. Coffee or alcohol work against vitamins, therefore they must not be used together.

IMPORTANT FACTS YOU SHOULD KNOW ABOUT VITAMINS

A vitamin is defined as an indispensable, essential, non-caloric, organic nutrient needed in tiny amounts in the daily diet. The role of the vitamin is to serve as a helper to the cell machinery, making it possible for nutrients to be digested, absorbed, metabolized and/or built into new body structure. Vitamins are not oxidized themselves, but they help to liberate energy from food for human use.

Today, more than 90 million adult Americans take vitamin supplements. Some of these people are taking extremely large doses in belief that the more vitamins you take, the more protection you get from disease. Each year increasing numbers of people report to hospitals for vitamin poisoning. Some vitamins are extremely harmful. Large doses of vitamin intake may damage the liver and kidneys. One should know that the human body needs very tiny amounts of vitamins to carry on the physiological processes. Daily consumption of fruits and vegetables can meet vitamin requirements. Since most people eat very little fruits and vegetables, they may need to take vitamin supplements, however we must be very careful not to overdose.

There is no difference between natural and synthetic vitamins. A cell picking up vitamins from the blood stream cannot tell the difference between vitamins derived from pills or from foods. Those who take vitamin supplements should take into consideration the following:

1. Never take vitamins without food. You gain no benefit. Vitamins only aid digestion, absorption and metabolism of foods; that is all.
2. Coffee, tea and alcohol have an anti-vitamin effect. If taken together, vitamins lose their beneficial effect.
3. Vitamins cannot satisfy hunger nor can they produce hunger.
4. There is no difference between synthetic vitamins and natural vitamins.
5. The intake of large dosages of vitamins are dangerous and can poison your body.

VITAMIN SUPPLEMENTS

I hope that you have read and learned a great deal about nutrition education from the information that I have provided in this book. Now you know more about vitamins, minerals, protein, fat, carbohydrates and their roles in health promotion. Since the foods we consume today are not 100 percent natural, we may need certain vitamin or mineral supplements. On that basis, I recommend taking some vitamin and mineral supplements to meet the needs of the body. There are two groups of vitamins which are very important:

Group A—The Antioxidant Vitamins. They include Vitamin A, Vitamin C and Vitamin E.

These vitamins are beneficial because:

1. They protect the immune system and prevent infection.
2. They prevent cancer and protect the tissue from damage caused by free radicals.
3. They slow down the aging process.

Recommended Supplements:

Vitamin A	10,000 I.U.
Vitamin C	500 Mg
Vitamin E	800 I..U.

Group B—These vitamins are involved in the production of energy. They include Folic Acid, Vitamin B1 and Vitamin B12.

Recommended Supplements:

Folic Acid	400 Mcg
Vitamin B1	50 Mg
Vitamin B12	50 Mg

In addition to vitamins, there are certain minerals that are essential for the normal functions of the body. They include:

1. Calcium—for the bones and muscles
2. Zinc—for hair, skin and protection against prostrate cancer
3. Chromium—for production of energy
4. Potassium—for prevention of water retention

Recommended Supplements:

Calcium	800 Mg
Chromium	200 Mg
Zinc	20 Mg
Potassium	100 Mg

CLASSIFICATION OF VITAMINS:

Vitamins are divided into two groups.
1. Water soluble
2. Fat soluble

Water soluble vitamins are soluble in water and they cannot be stored in the body. They must be supplied on a daily basis. Excessive amounts of these vitamins are excreted through the urine. On the other hand, fat soluble vitamins are only soluble in fat. They can be stored in the body. There is no need for daily intake. Excessive intake of these vitamins can be toxic and harmful and may cause liver damage.

The Fat Soluble Vitamins:

1. Vitamin A	(Retinal)
2. Vitamin D	(Calciferol)
3. Vitamin E	(Tocopherol)
4. Vitamin K	

The Water Soluble Vitamins:

1. Vitamin B1	(Thiamine)
2. Vitamin B2	(Riboflavin)
3. Niacin	(Nicotinic acid)
4. Vitamin B6	(Pyridoxine)
5. Folic Acid	
6. Pantothenic Acid	

7. Biotin
8. Vitamin B12   (Cobalamin)
9. Vitamin C

VITAMIN A

Vitamin A was the first fat soluble vitamin to be recognized. Two groups of research workers, McLean and Davis at the University of Wisconsin, and Mandel at Yale University made the discovery in 1913. They found that young animals became unhealthy and failed to grow on diets lacking natural fats. They also found that eyes become inflamed and infected but could be quickly relieved by the addition of a natural fat to their diets.

Functions:

1. Vision. Both day and night vision require Vitamin A. But night vision depends on the Vitamin A mechanism entirely. A deficiency in Vitamin A causes difficulty seeing in the dark. When there is Vitamin A deficiency, you cannot see the road after your eyes have been exposed to the headlights of an oncoming car.

2. Itching and Burning Eyes. Lack of Vitamin A causes burning and itching eyes. Eyelids become inflamed and eyeballs become painful.

3. Skin. Deficiency of Vitamin A affects the skin. The cells in the lower layers of the skin die and slough off. They plug oil sacs and pores, preventing oil from reaching the surface. The skin becomes so dry and rough that the entire body begins to itch. The roughness of the skin usually occurs first on the elbows, knees, buttocks and the backs of the upper arms.

4. Mucous Membrane. The mucous membrane protects the inside of the throat, nose, sinuses, middle ears, lungs, urinary tract and the gall bladder from infection. If the diet is adequate in Vitamin A, the mucous membrane continuously protects the body. The role of a mucous membrane is to secrete mucous to cover the cells, preventing

bacteria from reaching them. Bacteria cannot function in the mucous environment. They die.

5. Growth and Bone Development. Vitamin A is essential to the development of bone and teeth enamel. Lack of Vitamin A slows growth and development.

6. Immunity. Vitamin A deficiency increases susceptibility to bacterial, viral or parasitic infections. It is because of this observation and the fact that Vitamin A is important in maintaining the integrity of the mucous membrane that Vitamin A is known as the anti-infection vitamin. Without Vitamin A the barrier system against infection is gone.

7. Anti-Cancer. Several studies indicated that Vitamin A has a role in promoting normal functions of the epithelial cells and by doing that it prevents the development of malignancy in these cells. For this reason, Vitamin A is being used in humans to treat cancer, especially the cancers of the skin, lungs, breast and bladder.

Sources:

The leading dietary sources of Vitamin A are liver, eggs, whole milk, butter and cheese. Sources among vegetables are dark green, leafy and yellow vegetables such as collard, spinach, carrots, squash and sweet potatoes. Fruit sources include peaches, cantaloupe and melons.

Requirements:

The requirement of Vitamin A for men is 5000 I.U. per day. For women it is 4000 I.U. per day, but during pregnancy and lactation, the requirement increases to 6000 I.U. per day.

VITAMIN E

Vitamin E was discovered by Evans and Bishop in 1922 when they found that rats reared on a basic diet failed to reproduce until they were given a substance isolated from vegetable oil. After giving this substance, the rats produced robust offspring. This substance was given the name Vitamin E or anti-sterility vitamin. In 1936, it was chemically identified.

Functions:

1. Antioxidant. Vitamin E acts as an antioxidant. It serves to prevent unsaturated fatty acid from being destroyed in the body by oxygen. It also protects fatty like substances such as sex hormones and adrenal hormones from destruction.
2. Vitamin E prevents free radicals from damaging the cell membrane. Free radicals speed up the aging process in humans. Vitamin E, by destroying free radicals, slows down the aging process.
3. Vitamin E prevents anemia. Many red blood cells die everyday. To replace the dying cells, the body needs Vitamin E. Vitamin E is very important during pregnancy. Deficiency in pregnant women causes anemia in the newborn baby. During space flights, astronauts who spent more than eight days in space lost between 20 to 30 percent of their red blood cells. When they returned to earth they were extremely tired and their hearts so weakened that it puzzled their physicians. The reason discovered for these problems was due to the oxygen rich atmosphere which rapidly destroyed unsaturated fatty acid in the cells.
4. Vitamin E prevents blood clots. Vitamin E prevents the formation of a brown pigment produced by oxidation of unsaturated fatty acid by the presence of oxygen. These pigments prevent the production of an enzyme that dissolves the blood clot. This is the major problem in stroke, heart attack, phlebitis and varicose veins.

Sources:

Vitamin E is found in the following foods—nuts, liver, eggs, wheat breads, vegetable oils and green vegetables. Wheat germ oil is the richest source.

Deficiency:

Newborn babies low in Vitamin E will develop hemolytic anemia. This may be due to the feeding of formulas high in unsaturated fatty acids and iron. Formulas have a deficiency in Vitamin E, whereas human milk contains sufficient amounts of Vitamin E to meet the infants requirements. The major problem related to Vitamin E deficiency is muscle weakness, especially calf muscles become very painful during walking.

Requirements:

The allowance for infants is 200 I.U. per day. For adult males and females it is 400 I.U. per day. A diet high in polyunsaturated fat such as vegetable oils requires more Vitamin E.

ANTIOXIDANTS

More than a million Americans are diagnosed with cancer each year. In an effort to avoid this, people should eat more fiber and reduce the consumption of meat and fats. In recent years scientists have realized that fruits and vegetables are the best defense against cancer. Today, the hidden world of natural chemicals in edible plants is unfolding. There is an explosion of compelling and consistent data associating diets rich in fruits and vegetables with lower cancer risk. Data from 23 epidemiological studies clearly shows that a diet rich in fruits and vegetables slashed colon cancer by 40%. Another study shows that women who ate few fruits and vegetables had 25% higher breast cancer than women who consumed more fruits and vegetables. Evidence such as these have encouraged scientists to try and analyze just what it is about fruits and vegetables that have the ability to fight cancer. They believe that it is not vitamins and minerals or proteins that are protecting the body from cancer, but it is a biochemical substance called phytochemical.

When life began, plants were anaerobic. They lived in a world without oxygen. As they evolved they began to turn carbon dioxide into oxygen. They gradually polluted their own environment. In order to survive, plants were forced to develop chemicals (antioxidants) to defend against the unstable form of oxygen. These chemicals are called phytochemicals, many of which are brightly colored give plants their vivid colors. These colors are key parts of an antioxidant defense system. In addition to resisting oxidation, these substances fight against viral attack, harsh weather and other environmental forces. There are hundreds of phytochemicals that are classified in several groups by chemical names, by primary food sources and by anti-cancer action. Foods may contain numerous phytochemicals, each acting through one or more mechanisms.

Flavonoids

These are chemicals widely spread in fruits and vegetables. They reduce cancer risk by acting as antioxidants, blocking the action of carcinogens to cells by suppressing malignant changes in cells. They also interfere with the binding of hormones to cells, thus inhibiting cancer development.

Vitamin K

Vitamin K was discovered in 1935. Chickens fed on a ration adequate in all dietary essentials produced a severe hemorrhagic disease. When chickens were given hog liver, normal clotting time was restored. It was discovered that the hemorrhage was due to a lack of prothrombin, a compound required for a normal clotting of blood. This compound was called Vitamin K "Koagulation Vitamin".

Function:

Vitamin K has one major function. It is necessary for normal clotting of blood. A deficiency of Vitamin K is manifested by prolonging clotting time. Administration of Vitamin K to mothers prior to birth of newborn babies has reduced the incidence of hemorrhage among newborn infants. A deficiency of Vitamin K may occur when diets lack green vegetables. The growth of intestinal microorganisms is inhibited by using too much antibiotic medicine.

Sources:

There are two major sources of Vitamin K.

1. Ingested foods
2. Intestinal synthesis

Foods such as green vegetables, spinach, kale, broccoli, cabbage, lettuce and alfalfa are the richest sources of Vitamin K. Vitamin K is also found in tomatoes, liver, soybeans and eggs.

3. Bacterias in the intestinal tract produce Vitamin K, but excessive use of antibiotic medicine destroys these beneficial bacterias and produces Vitamin K deficiency.

Requirement:

No specific estimate of Vitamin K requirement has been made for humans, but 2 mg. of Vitamin K per day will correct Vitamin K deficiency in most cases. The suggested intake for adults is 70 mg. per day.

VITAMIN D

Vitamin D was discovered in 1930 and it was synthesized in 1936. The special role of this vitamin is to be sure that sufficient calcium is available in the blood that feeds the growing bone structure. It is also very important in the maintenance of the normal serum level of calcium and phosphorus. The most obvious sign of Vitamin D deficiency is the abnormality of bones. Examples are rickets and osteoporosic conditions in which calcium, when withdrawn from bones, causes the bones to lose their minerals and become porous, weak and easy to break. Some deafness can also be caused by Vitamin D deficiency because sound is transmitted along tiny ear bones to the brain. These bones also degenerate when there is not adequate Vitamin D in the body. Prolonged breast feeding without Vitamin D supplement or omission of milk from the diet of children can lead to rickets. In the old days, when there were no labor laws to govern child labor, a large number of children worked in the factories for long hours and did not receive any sunlight. The disease of rickets was more prevalent among these children. Rickets is a disease where bones, especially the bones of the legs, are not calcified completely, and are unable to support the weight of the body. As a result, the bones become bent, resembling a bow. For that reason it is called bow legs.

Requirement:

The daily requirement of Vitamin D is not necessary because the excesses are stored in the body. Vitamin D is extremely toxic. Special care must be taken in regard to the usage of this supplement. The toxicity symptoms are headache, diarrhea and nausea.

Sources:

The major sources of Vitamin D are egg yolks, liver, butter, and fish oils. In the United States, milk is fortified with Vitamin D, therefore milk can be a good source of this vitamin. The human body also makes Vitamin D when it is exposed to the sun. The sunlight converts the cholesterol contained in the skin into Vitamin D.

THE WATER SOLUBLE VITAMINS

THIAMINE

Thiamine is a water soluble vitamin and cannot be stored in the body. It requires daily intake. Thiamine in the body acts as a coenzyme. It releases energy from carbohydrates and traps energy. Cells can utilize that energy when they do work necessary for the body as a whole. Thiamine itself is not a source of energy, but it helps in the process of activating energy in food. This vitamin also plays an important role in the transmission of nerve impulses and efficiency of cardiac muscle. A deficiency in Thiamine causes nausea, severe fatigue, loss of appetite, abnormal heart beat, headache, insomnia, pain in the calf muscles, numbness in the feet and depression.

Requirement:

Since Thiamine cannot be stored in the body, it requires daily intake. Food containing Thiamine should be consumed on a daily basis. The requirement for adults is 2 mg. per day, but excessive alcohol intake increases the need for more of this vitamin.

Sources:
Lean pork, liver, yeast, legumes, and fresh green vegetables are the major sources of this vitamin.

Thiamine deficiency:
Thiamine deficiency causes weakness of eye movement, poor muscle coordination, memory loss, confusion and short attention span. People with high carbohydrate diets and infants fed by Thiamine deficient mothers can rapidly develop the acute symptoms of beriberi, a disease characterized by weakness of the legs, calf muscles and cramps. Walking becomes very difficult and heartbeat irregularities are experienced.

RIBOFLAVIN

Riboflavin is a coenzyme playing a vital role in the production of energy. It repairs damaged tissues. It also breaks down amino acids and fatty acids. A deficiency of this vitamin causes skin inflamation over the nose and eyes. It also causes cracks on the lips and in the corners of the mouth.

Requirements:
The daily requirement for adults is 2 mg. per day, but children who are in the process of growth need more of this vitamin—at least 4 mg. per day.

Sources:
Milk and milk products are the major sources of this vitamin. They provide half of the daily requirement. The other sources are dark green vegetables, nuts, seeds and organ meats.

Deficiency:
Eye problems, tissue damage and growth failure occur when the deficiency of Riboflavin occurs in the body. Skin inflammation near the

nose and eyes, cracks on the lips and corners of the mouth, swelling of the tongue, eye strain and headaches are among the symptoms.

NIACIN

Niacin is necessary for energy production. It was discovered in 1867 and its importance was not found until much later when the disease called pellagra was discovered. Pellagra is a skin disease caused by lack of Niacin in the diet. This disease sometimes was called rough skin disease and was occurring predominantly in the poor areas of Europe and in the southern section of the United States. After several years of research, it was found that the causes of the disease was based on a diet consisting of corn meal, pork fat and molasses. The key nutrient that was lacking in the diet of pellagra patients was an amino acid called tryptophan, which is found in lean meats. Pellagra is characterized by a disturbance of every tissue. Symptoms include weakness of the muscles, loss of appetite, diarrhea, a skin rash appearing on parts of the body exposed to the sun, confusion and memory loss.

Niacin Deficiency:

Niacin deficiency symptoms include weakness, fatigue, loss of appetite, indigestion, inflammation of the tongue, mouth and the digestive tract. Anemia and vomiting may occur after a few months of Niacin deficiency. If the deficiency continues, memory loss, dizziness and confusion develop.

VITAMIN B-6

Vitamin B6 or Pyridoxine is a water soluble vitamin. It cannot be stored in the body and it must be taken on a daily basis either by eating foods that contain this vitamin or by taking supplements. The vitamin was discovered in 1926.

Vitamin B6 plays a vital role in the formation of serotonin which controls the neurological activities of the brain. As a coenzyme, it converts tryptophan to Niacin. It also helps in the synthesizing of red blood cells. The blood glucose level is also regulated by Vitamin B6. Lack of B-6 causes depression, nervous irritation, impaired immune system, severe fatigue, skin disorders and water retention.

Requirement:

The daily requirement for adult men and women is 2 mg. per day. High intake of this vitamin may cause numbness of hands and feet.

Sources:

The major sources of this vitamin are green leafy vegetables, fruits, fish and meats.

Deficiency:

Lack of Vitamin B6 interferes with the production of two regulatory compounds in brain activity —serotonin and amino butyric acid. Both of these compounds control neurological conditions of people deficient in this vitamin. Lack of B-6 increases irritability that may progress to seizures. Vitamin B6 deficiency can cause anemia characterized by fatigue, lack of energy, water retention, and disturbance of sleeping patterns .These symptoms can be observed among Vitamin B6 deficient individuals.

FOLIC ACID

Folic acid is an anti-anemia vitamin and it is necessary for the production of red blood cells. It is not only necessary for production of the red cells, but it is responsible for their maturation as well. Without folic acid, red cells cannot be developed into functional cells to carry oxygen in the blood. Symptoms of folic acid deficiency are tiredness, shortness of breath, forgetfulness, sore tongue and diarrhea. These symptoms disappear when treated with folic acid.

Requirement:

The requirement for adult men and women is 2 mg. per day, but pregnant women need a little more. Lack of folic acid during pregnancy may leave mental defects in a newborn baby.

Sources:
Folic acid is found in green leafy vegetables, dairy products, organ meats and fresh fruits such as oranges and melons.

Deficiency:
When the level of folic acid decreases, changes occur in the production of red cells. In the bone marrow, as the number of cells decreases, the size of the red cells increase. These large cells are different in the total hemoglobin (iron) content. These cells cannot fulfill the work of regular red cells. Red cells carry oxygen from lungs to tissues and carbon dioxide away from tissues to lungs. As a result several symptoms develop. These symptoms include tiredness, diarrhea, sore tongue, shortness of breath, irritability and forgetfulness.

PANTOTHENIC ACID

This vitamin was discovered in 1938 and it is essential for metabolism of fat, protein and carbohydrate. It also plays a very important role in the function of the nervous system. Lack of this vitamin causes muscular weakness, cramps, numbness and prickling of the extremities. In the digestive system, lack of this vitamin may cause cancer of the colon and other digestive disorders.

Requirement:
Pantothenic acid is a water soluble vitamin and must be supplied daily. The requirement is 7 mg. per day for adult men and women.

Sources:
The major sources of this vitamin are legumes, nuts, fruits and poultry.

Deficiency:
The symptoms of deficiency include weakness, cramping, vomiting, insomnia, prickling and numbness of the extremities. These symptoms quickly disappear when pantothenic acid intake is normalized.

VITAMIN B12

Pernicious anemia was responsible for the death of many people before the discovery of Vitamin B12. In 1948, B12 was discovered and it saved the lives of thousands of people. It is essential for the formation of DNA, protection of the sheath surrounding nerves, and the production of red blood cells. Lack of this vitamin causes a specific disease called pernicious anemia. Pernicious anemia is characterized by the release of large, immature red blood cells from the bone marrow into the blood stream.

Requirement:
The daily requirement for adult men and women is 3 mg. per day.
Sources:
Vitamin B12 can only be found in foods of animal origin. No sources are available from plant foods. Meats such as pork, beef, poultry, seafood and dairy products are the major sources of this vitamin.
Deficiency:
Vitamin B12 deficiency causes pernicious anemia. It is characterized by large and immature red blood cells that develop in the bone marrow and enter the blood stream. These cells are not able to carry on the work of normal red cells. That is why pernicious anemia occurs. The characteristics of this form of anemia are weakness, paleness, depression, confusion and unsteadiness.

VITAMIN C

The scientific research on Vitamin C began in 1907 when two Norwegian scientists, Holst and Frolich produced scurvy, a deficiency disease associated with Vitamin C, in guinea pigs. The first experiment on humans was conducted by a British physician who was searching for a cure for scurvy. He divided his scurvy identified patients into four groups receiving vinegar, sulfuric acid, sea water, and lemon and oranges. The group receiving the lemon and oranges was cured within a short time. The other groups died. When the news arrived in England, the British Parliament ordered that all ships leaving England on long voyages must carry lime juice and that each sailor must receive lime juice daily. For that reason, the name "limey" was given to the British sailors. Vitamin C is a water soluble vitamin and it is not stored in the body. It requires daily intake. The excess of this vitamin is readily excreted. Vitamin C is an acid, and when combined with calcium, it produces kidney stones. Therefore, larger amounts of Vitamin C intake may contribute to the formation of kidney stones. Vitamin C is necessary for the building and maturation of bone matrix, cartilage, dentine, collagen and connective tissue. Vascular tissue and blood vessel walls are weakened without the cementing substance of Vitamin C to provide strong capillary walls.

Deficiency:

Vitamin C deficiency is characterized by fragile, easy rupture of capillaries with consequent tissue bleeding. Clinical conditions include easy bruising, easy bone fracture, poor wound healing, and bleeding gums with loosened teeth. Vitamin C plays a very important role in the production and maturation of red blood cells which are responsible for oxygen delivery to the entire tissues.

Requirement:

Vitamin C can be depleted by fever and infection, stress, injury, fracture and illness. Therefore people with stress, illness or pregnant women need to take more Vitamin C. The daily requirement is 60 mg. per day.

Sources:

The best sources of Vitamin C are citrus fruits and tomatoes, however cabbage, potatoes, green peppers, green vegetables, pineapple, broccoli and berries can provide a good source of this vitamin.

CHAPTER 11

MINERALS

The invention of the electric battery in the later part of the eighteenth century led Sir Humphrey Davey to the discovery of a number of minerals that are very important in nutrition. About 4 to 5 percent of our body weight is made up from minerals. The minerals of the body are classified into two groups.

1. Minerals that are required in relatively larger amounts in the body. These are called macro-minerals. They are:

   Calcium   Sulfur
   Potassium   Phosphorous
   Sodium   Magnesium

2. Minerals that are required in very small amounts. They are called trace minerals. These include the following:

   Iron
   Zinc
   Fluoride

Functions of Minerals:

1. Regulates fluid balance in the body
2. Maintains acid-base balance
3. Maintains nerve activities
4. Maintains muscular activities
5. Helps to promote growth

CALCIUM

The word calcium is derived from the Latin word "calx" which means chalk. Osborn and Mendel, two nutritionists, working in the laboratory, discovered that rats did not grow when there was a lack of calcium in their diets. They found out that the body needed calcium throughout life, especially during periods of growth, pregnancy and lactation.

Function:

1. It is necessary for the formation of bones and teeth
2. It plays an important role in blood clotting
3. It controls rhythmic beating of the heart
4. Contraction of the muscles are facilitated by calcium
5. It plays a major role in releasing energy for muscular activities
6. It is needed for nerve transmission and the release of neurotransmitters at the synaptic junctions.

Factors That Increase Calcium Absorption:

1. Vitamin D stimulates intestinal absorption of calcium
2. The hydrochloric acid secreted by the stomach improves calcium absorption
3. Lactose, the sugar in milk, enhances calcium absorption
4. Protein. Foods high in protein accelerate calcium absorption

Factors That Reduce The Absorption Of Calcium

1. A diet high in fat lowers the absorption of calcium
2. Vitamin D deficiency reduces calcium absorption
3. Oxalic acid that is found in certain vegetables such as spinach, Swiss chard and beets reduces the absorption of calcium
4. Emotional stress influences the efficiency of calcium absorption
5. Lack of exercise and especially lack of weight bearing exercises such as walking, jogging and weight lifting causes a reduction in calcium absorption
6. Long term use of drugs, such as diuretics, results in decreased calcium absorption

Sources:

Milk and milk products are the richest sources of calcium. If milk or milk products are not included in the daily diet, it would be impossible to obtain an adequate amount of calcium.

Requirements:

The calcium requirement is much higher during infancy than any other period of life. This higher requirement is due to the higher rate of growth during this period. The need for calcium also increases during pregnancy and lactation. Since calcium is associated with growth, many adults feel that they do not need it, but this is not true. Calcium is very important for the normal function of the body and replacement of daily bone loss. The recommendation to meet the daily requirement is 1200 mg. per day.

OSTEOPOROSIS

This is a bone disease which occurs especially among people over 50 years of age. It is a metabolic disorder which may be defined as a reduction in the amount of bone mass. With bone loss, the skeleton loses strength and it cannot stand physical stress. With a minimum of physical stress, a fracture may occur. The rate of this disorder is very high among women after menopause. Osteoporosis can be detected by measuring the thickness of long bone, especially the femur, by x-ray examination.

Causes Of Osteoporosis:

Osteoporosis is the result of a variety of factors:

1. Lack of calcium intake during periods of growth
2. Lack of absorption of calcium from the digestive system due to the aging process
3. Vitamin D deficiency decreases calcium absorption
4. Lack of exercise. Exercise plays a very important role in calcium metabolism, especially weight bearing exercises, such as walking,

jogging and weight training. Other exercises may develop cardio-vascular fitness, but will not help in bone development.

Osteoporosis does not occur suddenly in old age, but it develops over a long period of time. Individuals complete their bone development somewhere within their twenties. The amount of bone attained at this point is nutritionally and genetically determined. Research suggests that the rate of bone loss after the fourth decade of life is the same among all people. That would imply that a person having less bone mass at maturity is at a higher risk for the development of osteoporosis.

Estrogen

Estrogen regulates bone mass. After menopause, the level of estrogen declines in women. This reduction in estrogen reduces the rate of calcium metabolism and weakens the bones. It is very important to notice that taking large amounts of calcium after age 50 will not prevent osteoporosis. The bones of the body must be strengthened during early age when the body is growing, by regular exercise, calcium and Vitamin D intake, so that by the time a person reaches age 50 they will have a strong bone structure. Any calcium supplement must be accompanied by Vitamin D and exercise.

IODINE

A small amount of iodine is found in the human body, but its major role in human nutrition is well established. Iodine is part of the thyroid hormones. It regulates body temperature, metabolic rate and growth. The content of iodine found in food depends on the amount of iodine present in the soil where plants are grown or on which animals graze. Large amounts of iodine are found in the ocean, making seafood a good source of iodine. Since iodine is not uniformly distributed in the United States, the use of iodine salt is very advisable. When the blood level of iodine is low, the cells of the thyroid gland enlarge. This is due to the synthesis of a thyroid precursor, intended to trap as many particles of iodine as possible. If the gland enlarges until it is visible, it is called a goiter.

Symptoms of Iodine Deficiency:
1. A low level of iodine produces fatigue, depression and anxiety
2. Metabolic rate goes down as the level of iodine in the blood is lowered. As a result of low metabolic rate, the body weight goes up.
3. A low level of iodine also increases the level of blood cholesterol

Sources:
Iodine is found in the foods as well as in trace amounts in drinking water. Seafood such as clams, lobsters, oysters, sardines and other fish are major sources of iodine. Salt water fish contains 300 to 3000 micrograms of iodine. Fresh water fish has 20 to 40 micrograms of iodine. The iodine content of milk and eggs is determined by the iodine available in the diet of the animals. Iodine found in vegetables is contingent upon the amount of iodine found in the soil in which they were grown.

Requirement:
The National Research Council has suggested 15 mcg. per day. Pregnant or lactating women require about 25 to 50 mcg. respectively.

Deficiency:
1. Endemic to goiter
2. Enlargement of the thyroid gland
3. Low basal metabolism
4. Muscular weakness
5. Dry skin
6. High blood cholesterol

MAGNESIUM

The importance of magnesium has only recently been emphasized in the human body. Magnesium is found in bone and in soft tissue. The body contains about 20 to 28 grams of magnesium.

Function:

Magnesium is essential for the production and transfer of energy for protein synthesis, contraction of muscle and excitability in nerves. Magnesium and calcium may have an antagonistic relationship with each other. Magnesium acts as having a relaxation role and calcium as a simulator, therefore intake of these two minerals must be in balance. Magnesium deficiency is manifested by anorexia, growth failure and /or neuromuscular changes. It may also produce depression and muscular weakness. A deficiency in magnesium may develop by dietary inadequacy, use of diuretics, stress and alcoholism.

Requirement:

Recommendation by the National Research Council is 350 mg. per day for adult males and females. For pregnant and lactating women it is 450 mg. per day.

Sources:

Magnesium is abundant in nuts, legumes, cereal and dark green vegetables. Other sources are seafood and cocoa.

Deficiency:

1. Loss of appetite
2. Muscle tremors
3. Vomiting
4. Poor muscular coordination
5. Weariness

POTASSIUM

Potassium is one of the important electrolytes. It contributes, along with sodium to a normal blood pH level. It facilitates enzyme reactions related to the metabolism of protein, carbohydrate and formation of glycogen. The level of body potassium is related to the lean body weight (muscle mass). The sudden death that occurs during severe diarrhea or fasting are thought to be due to heart failure caused by potassium deficiency. Dehydration leads to potassium loss from inside the cells. It is especially dangerous because potassium loss from brain cells makes the victim unaware of the need for water. Because of this it is advisable not to take diuretics (water pills) as the water pills cause a significant potassium loss. Diuretics should be taken only under the supervision of a physician. Physicians who prescribe diuretics must tell the patient to eat potassium rich foods. Gradual potassium depletion can occur when a person sweats day after day, or from working in a hot environment. Such people should eat more potassium rich foods. Potassium tablets should not be used except under the direction of a physician. The deficiency of potassium may be manifested in such conditions as vomiting, diarrhea, muscle weakness, anorexia and edema (water retention).

Potassium Requirement:

Daily requirement is 50 to 150 mg. per day. People working in hot environments or athletes require more potassium.

Sources:

Major sources of potassium are fruits, especially pears, prunes, bananas and oranges. Legume sources include lima beans, pinto beans and kidney beans. Among the vegetables, potatoes, spinach, cabbage, cauliflower, broccoli and winter squash are rich in potassium.

Deficiency:

1. Lack of energy
2. Higher pulse rate
3. Abdominal bloating
4. Heart abnormality
5. Poor intestinal tone
6. Constipation

FLUORIDE

The body of an average man contains 26 grams of fluoride. The average daily intake by adults is 44 mg. The fluoride content of food varies according to the content of the soil in which it was grown. Fluoride deficiency may occur at fluoride concentrations of 2 to 7 ppm. and osteoporosis at 8 to 20 ppm. In some parts of the United States, such as in the Western United States, the water sometimes contains 10 to 45 ppm. of fluoride, causing children's teeth to develop with mottled enamel. The teeth of these children are extremely resistant to tooth decay. In other areas, such as in Michigan and New York, where fluoride is deficient in the water, the incident of dental decay is very high .One mg. of fluoride per liter of water produces a 60 to 70 percent reduction in tooth decay. Fluoride must be introduced to children at the early stages of life when teeth are forming. In many countries fluoride is added to the drinking water where the natural fluoride content is low.

ZINC

Zinc is known to be essential for more than 70 different enzymes. There are 1.4 to 2.3 grams of zinc in the body of an adult. The liver, pancreas, kidneys and bones have the largest concentration of zinc.

Functions:

Zinc deficiency is associated with many physiological functions including:

1. Reproductive system and growth.
2. Digestive system. It causes diarrhea.
3. It affects the immune system by making infection likely, including infection of the digestive tract.
4. Deficiency interferes with absorption and metabolism of Vitamin A and Folic Acid. Other problems associated with zinc deficiency are: night blindness, thyroid disturbance, wound healing, dry skin and alteration in taste and smell.

Requirements:
Recommended allowance for adults is 12 mg per day, but the RDA recommends 18 mg per day for adults and 5 to 6 mg additional during pregnancy. Excessive intake of zinc causes diarrhea, vomiting, anemia, dizziness and kidney failure.

Sources:
Animal products and legumes are good sources of zinc, such as liver, eggs and lean meat.

Deficiency:
1. Muscle tremor
2. Loss of hair
3. Impaired taste
4. Impaired smell
5. Slow wound healing
6. Infection
7. Mental depression

SODIUM

The existence of sodium has been known throughout history. It is a very important nutrient and necessary for all functions of the body. The distribution of water in the body depends on the location and concentration of sodium and potassium. Muscles and nerve activities are all regulated by sodium and potassium. The activities of the kidneys regulate the blood sodium level. If the level of blood sodium drops below the normal range it causes anxiety, fatigue and fast pulse rate. The level of blood sodium drops during vomiting, diarrhea and heavy sweating. On the other hand, if the blood sodium level goes up it causes water retention, high blood pressure and lack of energy. During heavy sweating, vomiting and extensive burn, both water and sodium must be replenished to prevent medical problems from occurring. If only water is provided, the blood concentration of sodium will drop and symptoms of water intoxication can occur such as headache, poor memory and weakness.

Sodium constitutes two percent of the total minerals in the body. It is involved in three major physiological functions:

1. Maintenance of normal water balance
2. Maintenance of acid-base balance in the body
3. Maintenance of normal nerve and muscular transmission activities

If the blood concentration of sodium rises, as it will after a person eats a salty meal, the thirst mechanism ensures that a person will desire to drink water until the water balance is adjusted. A high intake of sodium causes water retention in the body. The water retention not only causes fatigue, irritation and sleep disturbance, but it also causes higher blood pressure. High salt intake is very dangerous to pregnant women. It increases blood pressure and also causes problems for the newborn. Therefore, pregnant women should be told to restrict their salt intake throughout pregnancy. Low blood sodium has it's own serious problems as well. When the level of blood sodium drops, as during vomiting, heavy sweating and diarrhea, it causes muscular cramps, fatigue, rapid pulse and low blood pressure.

Requirements:

In the United States, the consumption of salt is very high. It is about 10 to 18 grams per day. The average recommended sodium intake is 4 to 6 grams per day. One reason for higher consumption of salt is that Americans use more processed foods such as prepackaged foods and foods sold in jars and cans which are very high in salt concentration.

CHROMIUM

The concentration of chromium is higher during infancy than other periods of life. Concentrations of chromium in the tissues decreases steadily with increasing age.

Functions:
Chromium plays a very important role in glucose metabolism.
Deficiency of Chromium:
1. Reduces the production of insulin
2. Lowers the production of energy from glucose
3. Causes diabetes
Sources:
Major sources of chromium are potato, vegetable oils and whole wheat products.
Requirement:
The requirement of chromium is 50 to 200 mcgs for normal adults.
Deficiency:
Chromium deficiency is characterized by inability to metabolize glucose, slow growth, lack of energy, fatigue and peripheral neuropathy. Chromium reduces the cholesterol ratio which is a protective index for the rate of cardiovascular diseases.

PHOSPHORUS

Phosphorus makes up one percent of the body weight and 85 percent of it is found with calcium in the bones and teeth. It is the chief compound that gives teeth and bone strength and rigidity. Phosphorus is also part of DNA, the genetic code material present in every cell in the body. It is necessary for growth and development of the tissues. Phosphorus is one of the essential minerals. It comprises 22 percent of the total minerals in the body. Most of phosphorus is located in the bones and teeth and the rest of this mineral is found in the extra-cellular fluid.
Functions:
This mineral has several important functions in the body.
1. It is a key component in the structure of cell membranes.
2. It plays an important role in the metabolic process involving protein, carbohydrate and fat, and also in the production of energy.

3. Phosphorus with calcium is necessary for nerve transmission and muscular contraction.

Sources:

Animal foods are the best sources of this mineral, such as meat, fish, poultry, milk and eggs. Phosphorus is also found in grains and cereal.

Requirements:

The daily requirement of phosphorus is almost the same as that of calcium for all age groups. It is 800 to 900 mg per day.

IRON

The role of iron in the blood seems to hold peculiar fascination for Americans. Television and newspapers are telling women that they must take iron everyday and that they need more iron than men. Historically, iron was discovered in the nineteenth century. It was thought that iron was part of human blood. Most of the iron in the body is a component of the proteins hemoglobin and myoglobin. Both these components carry oxygen in association with iron. They contain hemoglobin as the oxygen carrier in red cells and myoglobin as the receiver in the muscle cells. All cells use oxygen and nutrients to keep pathways open for the constant release of energy. The red cells shuttle between metabolizing tissues and lungs to bring in fresh oxygen supplies.

Functions:

Iron plays a very important role in the production of red blood cells. When the level of iron goes down the red cells will contain too little hemoglobin. They become unable to carry enough oxygen to meet the cells needs. Iron deficiency symptoms are:

1. Lack of energy, lack of sleep, emotional stress.
2. Low learning ability, lack of competence, short memory, poor attention span.
3. Dry and itchy skin.

4. Infection. Iron deficiency has been shown to reduce the bodies resistance.

5. Lack of iron causes general fatigue, anemia and pain in the bones.

Requirement:

The daily allowance for iron is 18 mg per day. For women it is a little more. It is important that iron should be obtained from food sources rather than through supplementation. Iron from fortified foods and from supplements is poorly absorbed even though they may contain as much as 50 mg of iron per day. Cooking utensils can enhance the amount of iron. The iron content of 100 grams of meat simmered in a glass dish is 3 mg, however when it is cooked in an iron skillet it becomes 8 mg. You can triple the iron content of a scrambled egg by cooking it in an iron pan. Food containing 25 mg of Vitamin C can double the amount of iron absorbed.

Deficiency:

Iron deficiency has been cited as the most common of all deficiency diseases in both developing and under developed countries. The groups considered the most frequently at risk are infants under two years of age, teenagers, pregnant women and the elderly. Iron deficiency manifests itself by the development of anemia. It can be corrected by consuming a diet rich in iron and by providing iron supplements in the form of ferrous sulfate or ferrous glutamate. Sulfate ferrous glutamate iron deficiency can be caused by loss of blood and degenerative diseases that interfere with iron absorption.

Factors that enhance iron absorption:

1. Vitamin C. The effects of Vitamin C on iron absorption is widely accepted. It is now recommended that iron be accompanied by the intake of Vitamin C.

2. Animal protein. Not all protein enhances the absorption of iron, only a cellular protein such as beef, pork, veal, lamb, liver, fish and cow's milk can enhance iron absorption.

3. Human milk. Infants retain more iron from human milk than from cow's milk or infant formula.
4. Calcium. The presence of an adequate amount of calcium in the diet helps to increase iron absorption.

Factors that Decrease Iron Absorption:

1. Lack of hydrochloric acid in the stomach.
2. Administration of alkaline substances such as antacids interfere with iron absorption.

Sources:

The richest sources of iron are liver and pork, with liver containing the highest amount and chicken liver containing the lowest amount. Other meat products such as organ meats and eggs are good sources of iron. Green leafy vegetables and dried fruits make a good contribution. The greener the vegetables, the higher the iron content.

MINERAL TOXICITY

Minerals can be extremely toxic and cause a serious problem to the body. Special attention must be given to the trace minerals. Mineral supplements exceeding 1.5 times the recommendation should be taken only under medical supervision.

Trace minerals most likely to cause toxicity are:

Iron: A large dosage of iron supplement can be life threatening. Iron pills and vitamin supplements that contain iron can poison children. Excessive iron deposited in tissues, causes severe liver and heart damage.

Zinc: A high dosage of zinc interferes with iron and copper absorption. A zinc supplement taken at three times its requirement reduces good cholesterol in the blood by 15 percent. By taking a zinc supplement you may be increasing you risk for developing heart disease.

Selenium: Over intake of selenium is associated with hair loss, weakness, rashes and cirrhosis of the liver.

Iodine: High intake of iodine disturbs the function of the thyroid gland. This can occur in people who eat a lot of seaweed. Seaweed is very high in iodine.

Fluoride: High fluoride intake can mottle teeth during their development. It also weakens the tooth structure.

CHAPTER 12

WATER

Water in the human body is like a river crossing through the arteries, capillaries and veins carrying a heavy load of nutrients and waste products. Water is in every part of the body including the cells, bones, tissues, skin and ligaments. From 55 to 65 percent of the body is made up from water. Water molecules are also found inside proteins, glycogen and in other macro molecules of the body, helping to form their structure. A little alteration in the water content of the body can cause dehydration, shock and death.

Functions: Water serves many functions:

1. Water serves as a building material for growth and repair in the body.
2. Water plays an important role in digestion, absorption and excretion.
3. It acts as a transport medium for nutrients and all body substances.
4. Water carries the metabolic waste produced in the cells and excretes it through the urine.
5. Fiber and cellulose in food absorbs water and aids in the elimination of fecal residue.
6. Water maintains body temperature.
7. Water acts as a lubrication in the joints. Without water, joints cannot function properly.

8. Water serves as a shock absorber inside the eyes, spinal cord, heart, kidneys and liver. It protects the vital organs of the body. The body can survive a deficiency of all other nutrients for a long time, but it can survive only a few days without water. This is because the body must excrete a minimum amount of water each day, carrying the waste products generated by metabolic process.

Water Balance: The water content of the fat free body weight remains fairly constant by homoeostatic regulations. This is a result of the interaction among antidiuretic hormones, the gastrointestinal tract, the kidneys and the brain. The amount of water taken in daily is equal to the amount of water loss.

Water Intake: Water intake is controlled by thirst sensation. The thirst control centers are located in the hypothalamus. Thirst is stimulated when the water volume of the body decreases or receptors in the great vessels are affected.

Sources of Water: Most adults consume 1.5 to 2 liters of water daily through drinks and foods, plus water from the oxidation of food in the body.

A. Daily fluid intake provides 500 to 1500 ml of water

B. Daily food intake provides 800 to 1000 ml of water

C. Cellular oxidation of foods provides 200 to 300 ml of water daily

Thirst and satiety govern water intake. When the blood is too concentrated it's solutes attract water out of the salivary glands and the mouth becomes dry. As a result you drink to wet your mouth. The brain center becomes involved because the hypothalamus also monitors the salt concentration of the blood. When the salt concentration of the blood is too high, the hypothalamus initiates impulses that stimulate drinking behavior.

Water elimination: There are four ways in which the body eliminates water.

1. Water is lost from the lungs as we expire air.

2. Water is lost from the kidneys as urine. Normally an adult excretes 600 to 1600 ml of urine per day.

3. Water is lost through perspiration.

4. Water is lost through the bowel in the feces.

Abnormal water loss occurs through vomiting, diarrhea and hemorrhages. The body has no place to store water. Water must be replaced on a daily basis in order to maintain a healthy water balance.

Water Requirement: According to the Food and Nutrition Board, a daily water intake of 2.5 liters or 3 quarts of water is needed to carry on the essential activities of the body. Special attention should be given to adults or infants who are on protein diets, to people in hot environments or to those who have high fever and/or diarrhea.

CHAPTER 13

NUTRITIONAL DEFICIENCY DISEASES

DIABETES

Diabetes is one of the major diseases in the United States. More than 500,000 new cases are diagnosed each year. The yearly medical cost of this disease is more than 20 billion dollars. Diabetes is a disorder in which not enough insulin is produced within the body to move the glucose into the cell and use it for energy. As a result of insufficient insulin, the blood sugar rises. There are two major types of diabetes:

1. Insulin Dependent
2. Non-insulin Dependent

Insulin Dependent: In insulin dependent diabetes, the pancreas does not make insulin. Without insulin, the body cannot utilize the sugar and must try to use fat for energy. Combustion of fat results in an acid waste called Ketosis. As ketones build up in the blood supply, a serious metabolic condition known as Ketoacidosis occurs. If this condition is not treated it may result in death. This type of diabetes usually occurs in young children and is called Juvenile Onset Diabetes. Only 10 percent of all incidences of diabetes belongs to this group.

Non-Insulin Dependent: In non-insulin dependent diabetes, the pancreas makes some insulin, but it is an insufficient amount. Those having this type of diabetes still require some insulin from outside sources for normalizing the blood sugar. Of all the cases of diabetes, 85 percent are non-insulin dependent. Most of the non-insulin dependent cases occur after age 20 as a result of overeating, lack of exercise and gaining weight. Excessive amounts of body fat reduces the efficiency of insulin in the body.

Symptoms of Diabetes:

1. Frequent urination
2. Extreme hunger
3. Thirst
4. Blurred vision
5. Easy tiring
6. Drowsiness

Treatment:

1. A high fiber diet. Consumption of more fresh vegetables, fruits, legumes (beans, peas, lentils) and complex carbohydrates. The fiber found in these foods reduces insulin requirements and lowers fasting blood sugar and triglycerides.
2. Reduction of high fat foods. These include the following items: bacon, salad dressing, fried foods, cold cuts, alcohol, gravy, nuts, salt and non-complex carbohydrates (cakes, cookies, pastry and sugar products).

HYPOGLYCEMIA

Hypoglycemia is a low blood sugar that is related to excessive production of insulin.

Treatment:

Do not consume the following foods.

Pastries	Coffee
Soft Drinks	Sugar Products

Eat six small meals per day. Meals must include carbohydrates and proteins.

ASTHMA

It is the inflammation of the windpipe which can be caused by MSG, shell fish and additives in foods.

Treatment:

Avoid-

Cheese   Wine

Vinegar   Oranges

Shrimp   Gelatin

MSG

GOUT

It is caused by high uric acid in the blood through a high intake of beans, shellfish and red meat.

Treatment:

Avoid-

1. Beans, peas, spinach, mushrooms, lentils and asparagus
2. Pork, shellfish and red meat

Consume More-

1. Carbohydrate rich foods such as rice, bread, potato and pasta
2. Eggs, cheese and fruits
3. Drink more water

CONSTIPATION

Constipation is a problem of evacuation of the bowel, which is caused by slow movement of the feces through the large intestine. During a prolonged stay in the colon, the feces becomes dry and hard as the water content of the feces is increasingly absorbed. The food we eat plays a very important role in the movement of fecal materials. Foods high in fiber such as fruits, vegetables, whole wheat breads, rice and potatoes absorb water along the intestinal tract, thereby producing bulk and stimulating defecation. It is important that a person should have a daily bowel movement so that the digestive system stays clean and prevents the growth of bacteria.

Causes of Constipation:

1. Lack of exercise is an important factor in constipation. Exercise stimulates the intestinal muscles and strengthens them so that when the wall of the digestive tract contracts it produces a strong force and forces the residue down facilitating the process of defecation.
2. Another cause of constipation is insufficient water intake. Water is absorbed by food residue and produces a soft and bulky feces. Such residue can be moved easier down the tract. Therefore it is important that each person take at least four glasses of water per day.
3. Emotional stress. Emotional stress causes constriction of the blood vessels and spasms of the muscles around the large intestine. As a result the peristalsis movement slows down and the feces becomes dry and hard. This contributes to constipation.

Treatment:

1. Adequate water intake, about 3 to 4 glasses of water per day.
2. Participation in daily exercise. An exercise program should be 20 to 30 minutes of jogging or walking at least 5 times per week.
3. More fruits, vegetables, rice, legumes and whole wheat bread should be consumed.
4. Stress reduction. You may achieve this by becoming involved in meditation or some form of a hobby.

ACNE

It is caused by additives in the foods.

Treatment:

1. Wash face with warm water 5 times per day.
2. Take Vitamins A (20,000 I.U.), Vitamin C (1000 mg) and B Complex.
3. Eat more fresh fruits.

Do not use—
1. Cosmetics
2. Food or beverages sold in cans, bottles or jars.

SPASTIC COLON

Spastic colon is a common disorder of an unknown cause that does not appear to be any organic abnormality. It is the result of over stimulation of the intestinal nerve endings that cause irregular contraction of the bowel. There is a loss of rectal sensitivity which can cause either rapid transit through the bowel or constipation. It is usually accompanied by nausea, constipation or diarrhea, which may alternate. Because of the spasms, the mass moves more irregularly along the intestinal tract.

Causes: The causes of spastic colon are related to:
1. Emotional upset or a prolonged period of stress.
2. Excessive use of laxatives.
3. Excessive use of coffee or tea
4. Excessive use of tobacco
5. Excessive use of alcohol
6. Frequent use of antibiotics
7. Lack of regular sleep or rest

Symptoms: Symptoms of a spastic colon are-
1. Heartburn
2. Full feeling
3. Flatulence
4. Severe cramping and pain

Prevention:
1. A high fiber diet is recommended which will add bulk to the stool, relieve constipation and the pressure within the colon walls.
2. Low fat diet.

POOR CIRCULATION

It is caused by lack of exercise, weight gain and a high fat diet.
Treatment:
1. Exercise
2. Low fat diet
3. Weight Loss
4. Vitamin E (800 I.U.)
5. Folic Acid (400 mcg)

DIARRHEA

Diarrhea is the occurrence of frequent liquid stools. It is a symptom, not a disease. The passage of food through the intestinal tract is abnormally rapid. The residue passes through the colon so quickly that there is no chance for the fluid to be absorbed.

Classification:
There are two types of diarrhea.
1. Functional
2. Organic

Functional diarrhea is less severe and it may occur in any normal healthy person.

Causes: Some of the major causes of functional diarrhea.
1. Overeating
2. Eating the wrong foods
3. Fermentation caused by incomplete digestion
4. Nervous tension
5. Drinking too much coffee

Organic Diarrhea is usually caused by external poison, such as food poisoning or parasites. Sometimes it may be caused by enzyme deficiency that results in impaired digestion and absorption.

Treatment: In both cases of diarrhea, nutritional treatment is the same.
1. Provide a diet which leaves little residue.
2. In severe cases lasting 12 to 24 hours, fasting is essential to provide rest to the digestive tract.
3. Replacement of the fluid and electrolytes.

After 12 hours, simple foods such as dry toast and tea are given. Scraped raw apple or applesauce may be given every 4 hours. Vitamin B, Vitamin C and fruit juice should be given. When diarrhea stops, regular food should be taken gradually.

DIET AND TUMORS

The link between diet and tumors is very strong. Tumors do not appear out of nowhere. It takes years to produce a tumor. First, the process starts when something alters the genetic makeup of cells. Chemicals, viruses and radiation can damage cells, but the most important damaging agent of all is oxygen. In all activities we do, we generate reactive oxygen molecules called free radicals. These free radicals bounce around cells and steal electrons from molecules and consequently damage the DNA of the cells.

In the beginning of life, plants were anaerobic. They lived in a world free of oxygen. As they evolved, they began turning carbon dioxide into oxygen. By doing so, they polluted their environment with free oxygen which threatened their existence. In order to survive, they were forced to develop defenses against free oxygen. Plants began to produce a variety of colors: red, green, yellow, orange, purple and white. These colors were called phytochemicals which gave plants their vivid hues.

Phytochemicals are key parts of the antioxidant defense system. In addition to resisting oxidation, they guard against viral attack and harsh climate. The variety of colors that you find in fruits and vegetables are the colors that plants have produced to fight against free radicals, which are known to cause tumors. Since the consumption of fruits and vegetables have declined during the past 50 years, the cancer rate has climbed significantly. The American Cancer Institute concluded that poor eating habits are responsible for the high rate of cancer in the United States.

In order to combat cancer, we must do the following:

1. Increase the consumption of a variety of fruits, such as oranges, bananas, pears, apples and other fruits having different colors.
2. Increase the consumption of vegetables, such as kale, spinach, cabbage, tomatoes, eggplant, cucumber, squash, onion, peppers and other color varieties.

Each of these vegetables and fruits provide a strong shield against tumors. It is very important that we should include a variety of fruits and vegetables in our daily diet.

CHAPTER 14

LIST OF RECIPES

All Vegetables
Baked Flounder
Baked Shrimp
Calamari
Baked Veal Cutlet
Chicken and Veggies
Chicken Cutlet
Chicken Delight
Chicken La Bo
Chicken La Duma
Chicken La Shabo
Chicken La Supreme
Diabetic Vegetables
Dutchess's Dinner
Egg Omelet
Fish La Chanta
Fish La Dimarka
Grilled Chicken Breast
High Vegetable Diet
Hudson Delight
Hudson Salad Dressing
Hudson Scampi
La Fish

Liver La France
Microwave Chicken
Microwave Fish or Shrimp
Microwave Omelet
Oriental Supreme
Salad
Scallops Du Pan
Shrimp Dinner
Shrimp Salad Delight
Stuffed Flounder
Stuffed Pepper
Tooshi's Combo
Tooshi's Diabetic Soup
Tooshi's Dinner
Tooshi's Pilaf
Tooshi's Sauce
Tooshi's Shish-Ka-Bob
Tooshi's Soup
Tooshi's Stew
Vegetarian Dinner
Vegetarian II
Veggie Shrimp
Yuppie's Delight

ALL VEGETABLES

INGREDIENTS:
Two tablespoons grated cheese
Eggplant, zucchini, mushroom, garlic, broccoli, green pepper, tomato, any green leafy vegetables.
One potato
Seasonings: Onion, garlic powder, fresh red pepper
One cup water
DIRECTIONS:
1. Slice all vegetables and dice the potato
2. Add vegetables to a deep pot, add water and seasonings
3. Cook for 10 minutes
4. Drain and arrange vegetables on a dinner plate
5. Add grated cheese and serve

BAKED FLOUNDER

INGREDIENTS:
Six ounces flounder
Half cup each spinach and broccoli
One tomato
Five mushrooms
One fresh garlic (whole clove)
One fresh lemon
One teaspoon corn oil
Spices you like (no salt)
DIRECTIONS:
1. Preheat oven to 400
2. Place fish on aluminum foil. Add corn oil and spices
3. Slice lemon and place over fish

4. Chop all vegetables and add to the fish, wrap foil tightly
5. Cook 20 minutes and serve

BAKED SHRIMP

INGREDIENTS:
Six ounces shrimp
Two tomatoes
Cabbage, broccoli or spinach
Five mushrooms
One fresh lemon
One teaspoon corn oil
Seasonings: Onion and garlic powder, oregano
DIRECTIONS:
1. Preheat oven to 400.
2. Place shrimp in aluminum foil and place vegetables around shrimp
3. Add seasonings and corn oil. Place slices of lemon over the shrimp
4. Wrap foil tightly and bake 20 minutes, serve.

BAKED VEAL CUTLET

INGREDIENTS:
Six ounces veal cutlet
One or two tomatoes
Five mushrooms
Select either broccoli, cabbage or spinach
½ fresh lemon
One teaspoon corn oil
Spices you like: provided no salt

DIRECTIONS:
1. Preheat oven to 400.
2. Place veal cutlet onto a sheet of aluminum foil with all vegetables around the cutlet
3. Add corn oil and seasonings you like
4. Slice lemon and place over the veal
5. Wrap tightly, cook 20-25 minutes and serve.

CALAMARI

INGREDIENTS:
One teaspoon crushed garlic
Two teaspoons chopped ginger
Two tomatoes
One teaspoon parsley
Six ounces calamari
One teaspoon olive oil—1st frying pan
One teaspoon olive oil—2nd frying pan
Spices—pepper, onion powder
DIRECTIONS:
1. Heat the 1st frying pan with a teaspoon olive oil and add chopped garlic. Brown it.
2. Add ginger and crushed tomatoes. Cook for 6 minutes. Mix well.
3. Heat the 2nd frying pan with a ½ cup of water. Add calamari. Cook for 10 minutes.
4. Drain water. Add the contents of the first pan to the second pan.
5. Add spices, parsley, one teaspoon olive oil and mix well. Cook 5 minutes and serve.

CHICKEN AND VEGGIES

INGREDIENTS:
One chicken leg or three chicken drums
Green leafy vegetables, broccoli, zucchini, cabbage, cauliflower
Seasonings—garlic, onion powder, red pepper
A teaspoon corn oil
DIRECTIONS:
1. Remove the skin of the chicken, add seasonings. Bake 20 minutes at 400.
2. Steam all vegetables with a teaspoon corn oil and seasonings.
3. Serve over chicken.

CHICKEN CUTLET

INGREDIENTS:
Six ounces chicken cutlet
Three tablespoons orange juice
Spices—onion and garlic powder, red or black pepper
Select any of the following vegetables:

cabbage	peppers	broccoli
zucchini	cauliflower	asparagus

DIRECTIONS:
1. Place chicken cutlet in a baking dish
2. Combine spices and orange juice in a mixing bowl
3. Brush ½ of the mixture over the cutlet and bake at 400 for 10—12 minutes.
4. Turn cutlet over, brush on remaining mixture, add vegetables to baking dish
5. Return to oven. Cook another 8—10 minutes and serve.

CHICKEN DELIGHT

INGREDIENTS:
Two tomatoes
Four mushrooms
One clove garlic
6 oz. chicken cutlet
One tablespoon corn oil
DIRECTIONS:
1. Cut chicken cutlet into small cubes and cook in medium fry pan with ½ cup of water for 6—8 minutes.
2. Drain water. Cook another 3 minutes or until chicken is browned.
3. Add teaspoon corn oil, stir, cook another minute. Remove from heat.
4. Chop tomato, mushroom and garlic. Place into a second frying pan. Cook until all juice comes out of tomatoes and it becomes a sauce
5. Add chicken cutlet from 1st pan to the sauce, mix well, cook another 2—3 minutes and serve.

CHICKEN LA BO

INGREDIENTS:
6 oz. chicken cutlet
One teaspoon corn oil
One tablespoon grated cheese
½ cup broccoli
½ cup chopped string beans
DIRECTIONS:
1. Place all ingredients in a microwave dish
2. Brush a teaspoon corn oil over chicken
3. Cook 10—12 minutes on high
4. Add tablespoon grated cheese as a topping and serve

CHICKEN LA DUMA

INGREDIENTS:
6 oz chicken or turkey cutlet
Two tomatoes
One fresh garlic
Six mushrooms
One tablespoon corn oil
One cup water
Spices—onion and garlic powder, oregano
DIRECTIONS:
1. Put the cutlet on a frying pan with 1 cup water. Cover and cook 10 minutes.
2. Remove lid. Drain water. Add tablespoon corn oil.
3. Cook the cutlet on both sides until browned.
4. Chop all vegetables, add to cutlet. Cover and cook 6—8 minutes and serve.

CHICKEN LA SHABO

INGREDIENTS:
6 oz chicken cutlet
Half cup each broccoli and spinach
5 mushrooms
One clove garlic
1/4 fresh orange
Teaspoon corn oil
Spices—onion and garlic powder, oregano
DIRECTIONS:
1. Preheat oven to 400. Rub a teaspoon corn oil onto aluminum foil.
2. Add cutlet, orange wedges and spices.

3. Cut vegetables and arrange around the cutlet.

4. Wrap foil tightly. Bake 20-25 minutes and serve.

CHICKEN LA SUPREME

INGREDIENTS:

4 oz chicken cutlet

1/4 cup wine

2 tablespoons grated cheese

½ cup each mushroom, tomato and broccoli

Spices—onion and garlic powder

DIRECTIONS:

1. Preheat oven to 350.

2. Place cutlet in center of baking dish.

3. Add wine, grated cheese and spices over the cutlet.

4. Cover and bake 20—25 minute. Serve with steamed vegetables.

DIABETIC VEGETABLES

INGREDIENTS:

Kidney beans	Cabbage	Onion
Lentils	Garlic Clove	Tomato

One tablespoon corn oil

½ Cup water

Spices—onion and garlic powder

DIRECTIONS:

* Soak the beans and lentils at least 10 hours prior to cooking

1. Cook the beans and lentils in ½ cup of water for 8—10 minutes.

2. Chop vegetables, add to the beans and lentils.

3. Drain off water. Add chopped tomato.

4. Cook on low another 3—4 minutes and serve over baked chicken or fish.

*You may substitute canned beans or lentils provided you rinse and drain the beans first.

DUTCHESS'S DINNER

INGREDIENTS:
One medium potato
1/4 eggplant
2 tomatoes
5 mushrooms
½ zucchini
One teaspoon corn oil
Spices—oregano, onion and garlic powder
One tablespoon grated cheese
DIRECTIONS:
1. Add one teaspoon corn oil and one cup water to a deep pot.
2. Cut potato into cubes, add to pot. Boil for 6 minutes.
3. Cut and add all vegetables. Cook another 5 minutes over medium heat.
4. Drain water, add cheese and serve.

EGG OMELET

INGREDIENTS:
2 tomatoes
6 mushrooms
½ clove garlic
One teaspoon corn oil
Two eggs

Spices you like
One tablespoon grated cheese
DIRECTIONS:
1. Add teaspoon corn oil to a frying pan.
2. Chop and add all vegetables and spices.
3. Cover and cook over medium heat 6—8 minutes until all juice comes out of tomatoes and it becomes a sauce. Add cheese.
4. Add two eggs, mix well.
5. Cover and cook another 6 minutes and serve.

FISH LA CHANTA

INGREDIENTS:
6 oz flounder
2 tomatoes
One fresh garlic
6 mushrooms
One teaspoon corn oil
½ cup water
Spices—onion and garlic powder, oregano
DIRECTIONS:
1. Place the flounder in a frying pan with ½ cup water. Cover and cook 10 minutes.
2. Drain water, add corn oil.
3. Add chopped vegetables to the flounder.
4. Cover pan and simmer 6—8 minutes and serve.

FISH LA DIMARKA

INGREDIENTS:
6 oz flounder
6 fresh mushrooms

One clove garlic
2 tomatoes
½ fresh lemon
Spices you like
½ cup wine
DIRECTIONS:
1. Preheat oven to 400.
2. Place flounder in a baking dish.
3. Add teaspoon corn oil and ½ cup wine to the dish, cover with foil.
4. Cook 6—8 minutes.
5. Turn fish over. Add chopped mushroom, tomato and garlic.
6. Cook another 8 minutes and serve.

GRILLED CHICKEN BREAST

INGREDIENTS:
One split chicken breast
Fresh green vegetables (spinach, cabbage, broccoli)
One teaspoon corn oil
Spices—lemon, pepper, garlic powder
DIRECTIONS:
1. Remove skin from chicken. Place aluminum foil on grill, place chicken on foil.
2. Steam or boil the vegetables together.
3. Drain the vegetables.
4. Add corn oil and spices to vegetables. Let stand 1 minute.
5. Serve over grilled chicken.

HIGH VEGETABLE DIET

INGREDIENTS:

Onion   Garlic

Broccoli   Cabbage   Potato

1/4 cup barley

1/4 cup lentils

One tablespoon corn oil

One cup water

Spices you like

DIRECTIONS:

1. Place the barley, lentils and chopped potato in a deep pan. Add water and corn oil.

2. Cover and cook 10—12 minutes.

3. Chop and add remaining vegetables. Mix well.

4. Cover and cook another 6—8 minutes.

5. Drain off water. Serve with baked fish or chicken.

HUDSON DELIGHT

INGREDIENTS:

6 oz chicken cutlet

½ cup each broccoli, mushroom, spinach

One clove garlic

3 to 4 tablespoons Tooshi's Sauce

Spices you like

DIRECTIONS:

1. Place cutlet onto aluminum foil and arrange vegetables around the cutlet.

2. Add 3 to 4 tablespoons Tooshi's Sauce to chicken and add spices.

3. Wrap foil tightly, bake at 350 for 20 minutes and serve.

HUDSON SALAD DRESSING

INGREDIENTS:
1/3 cup vinegar
1/3 cup corn oil
1/3 cup lemon juice
Onion and garlic powder
Pepper
DIRECTIONS:
1. Combine all ingredients into a container, shake well.
2. Chill before using over salad.
3. Use no more than one tablespoon per serving.

HUDSON SCAMPI

INGREDIENTS:
6 large shrimp
½ chopped onion
3 cloves garlic
One teaspoon corn oil
One tablespoon fresh squeezed lemon
½ teaspoon paprika
1/4 cup water
DIRECTIONS:
1. Place all ingredients in a baking dish. Preheat oven to 350.
2. Bake 10—12 minutes. Remove from oven and stir ingredients.
3. Resume baking another 10—12 minutes.
4. Serve with tossed salad.

LA FISH

INGREDIENTS:
6 oz flounder
½ cup dry wine
Tablespoon crushed garlic
One medium tomato
One diced onion
4 mushrooms
Chopped parsley
½ tablespoon lemon juice
DIRECTIONS:
1. Add ½ cup wine to a frying pan. Bring to a boil.
2. Add flounder, onion, garlic and lemon juice.
3. Cover pan, saute fish on both sides for total of 8 minutes.
4. Add mushroom, tomato, parsley.
5. Cook another 6—8 minutes and serve.

LIVER LA FRANCE

INGREDIENTS:
4 oz beef or chicken liver
One onion
5 mushroom
One fresh garlic
2 tomatoes
½ tablespoon corn oil
Spices you like
DIRECTIONS:
1. Cover and cook liver in a frying pan with ½ cup water for 10 minutes.
2. Drain off water, add onions and corn oil, mix well.

3. Cook another 4—5 minutes or until onions become browned.

4. Add chopped tomato, mushroom and garlic, mix well.

5. Cover and cook another 6—8 minutes and serve.

MICROWAVE CHICKEN

INGREDIENTS:
6 oz chicken cutlet
5 mushrooms
One tomato
Broccoli
Green and red peppers
Two tablespoons of white wine
Spices you like
DIRECTIONS:
1. Add 2 tablespoons wine to a cooking dish. Slice cutlet into filets.
2. Place filets into dish, add spices.
3. Cut all vegetables and arrange around chicken.
4. Cover dish. Cook on high approximately 8 minutes and serve.

MICROWAVE FISH OR SHRIMP

INGREDIENTS:
6 oz fish or shrimp
One fresh lemon
One tomato

Broccoli and cauliflower
4 mushrooms
One fresh garlic
2 tablespoons of white wine
Spices you like

DIRECTIONS:
1. Add 2 tablespoons wine to a cooking dish, add fish or shrimp.
2. Add spices and slices of lemon over the fish or shrimp.
3. Arrange vegetables around the fish or shrimp.
4. Cover and cook 10—12 minutes and serve.

MICROWAVE OMELET

INGREDIENTS:
2 eggs
2 tomatoes
6 mushrooms
One fresh garlic
1 cup chopped spinach
One teaspoon corn oil
Spices you like
DIRECTIONS:
1. Chop all vegetables and set aside.
2. Break two eggs into cooking dish, add spices and corn oil, Mix well.
3. Add vegetables, mix well. Cover the dish.
4. Set in microwave and cook 2 minutes on high.
5. Remove dish, stir ingredients, cook on high another 2—3 minutes and serve.

ORIENTAL SUPREME

INGREDIENTS:
½ cup dry rice
½ zucchini
2 tomatoes
5 mushrooms

1/4 eggplant
One teaspoon corn oil
Spices you like

DIRECTIONS:
1. Add ½ cup rice to sauce pan, add enough water so that water is one inch above the rice.
2. Cover and cook over high heat until rice boils.
3. Lower the heat, stir well, continue cooking 10 minutes longer.
4. Remove pan from stove, set in cold water so that rice will not stick to pan.
5. In a separate pan, place all chopped vegetables. Add water, corn oil and spices.
6. Boil five minutes, drain water and serve over rice.

SALAD

INGREDIENTS:
A good salad should contain the following vegetables

cabbage	radish	Romaine lettuce
carrot	onion	spinach
cucumber	peppers	tomato

Salad plays a very important role in our daily diet. It provides an abundance of fiber, vitamins and minerals. Most of the vitamins in our food is destroyed by heat. Salad is not exposed to heat and is therefore a rich source of vitamins and minerals. These vegetables are very low in calories. You can eat as much as you like. The primary problem with salad involves the commercial dressings. The best dressing is vinegar or Tooshi's Dressing. If you cannot use these, then ½ tablespoon of any low-fat commercial salad dressing is permissible.

SCALLOPS DU PAN

INGREDIENTS:
6 oz scallops
2 tomatoes
One fresh garlic
One cup chopped spinach
One cup chopped mushroom
One teaspoon corn oil
½ cup water
Spices you like
DIRECTIONS:
1. Add ½ cup water in a frying pan. Bring to boil.
2. Add scallops, lower heat, cover and cook 8—10 minutes.
3. Remove lid, drain water.
4. Add chopped vegetables and corn oil. Stir.
5. Cover and cook 6—8 minutes and serve.

SHRIMP DINNER

INGREDIENTS:
6 medium shrimp
2 tomatoes
One fresh garlic
6 mushrooms
One teaspoon corn oil
½ cup water
Spices you like (red/black pepper, oregano, garlic powder)
DIRECTIONS:
1. Add ½ cup water to frying pan, bring to boil.
2. Add shrimp, cover and cook 8—10 minutes over high heat.

3. Remove cover, drain water, add corn oil. Stir.

4. Add mushrooms, tomato, and garlic.

5. Lower heat, cover and cook another 5—6 minutes and serve.

SHRIMP SALAD DELIGHT

INGREDIENTS:
6 shrimp
One tomato
½ green pepper
4 radishes
Romaine Lettuce
½ cucumber
Lemon juice and vinegar
DIRECTIONS:
1. Chop shrimp into bite sized pieces.
2. Boil the shrimp 6—8 minutes.
3. Drain water. Chill in lemon and vinegar.
4. Mix with salad vegetables, add spices and serve.

STUFFED FLOUNDER

INGREDIENTS:
4 flounder fillets
One cup chopped spinach
One cup chopped scallion
1/4 chopped onion
One tablespoon lemon
1/4 cup dry wine
½ teaspoon paprika

DIRECTIONS:
1. Place flounder into a baking dish.
2. Spread chopped spinach, scallion and onion over each slice.
3. Roll up each fillet and fasten with toothpick.
4. Pour wine and lemon juice over the fillets.
5. Sprinkle with paprika.
6. Bake at 350 for 20—25 minutes and serve.

STUFFED PEPPERS

INGREDIENTS:
2 oz ground beef
½ chopped onion
2 chopped mushrooms
½ whole garlic
One chopped tomato
2 large green peppers
One teaspoon grated cheese
DIRECTIONS:
1. Cook beef in a sauce pan with ½ cup water for 8—10 minutes.
2. Drain water.
3. Chop all vegetables, add to the beef.
4. Mix well, cook another 6 to 7 minutes.
5. Slice peppers in two parts and stuff them with the vegetable and beef mixture.
6. Hold peppers together with toothpicks. Bake in oven at 350 for 15 minutes and serve.

TOOSHI'S COMBO

INGREDIENTS:
4 to 6 oz lean beef
Half cup each broccoli, mushroom, spinach, string beans
One fresh garlic
3 to 4 tablespoons Tooshi's Sauce
Spices you like
DIRECTIONS:
1. Slice beef into thin strips. Place onto aluminum foil.
2. Place vegetables around the beef.
3. Add 3 to 4 tablespoons of Tooshi's Sauce.
4. Place in oven. Bake at 350 for 20 minutes and serve.

TOOSHI'S DIABETIC SOUP

INGREDIENTS:

| kidney beans | lentils | onion |
| garlic | tomato | broccoli |

1/4 pound chicken cutlet
Tablespoon corn oil
Spices—bay leaf, basil, onion and garlic powder
DIRECTIONS:
*Soak dry kidney beans and lentils 10 hours before making soup.
1. Cook chicken in ½ cup water. Add 1 tablespoon corn oil and spices.
2. Chop the vegetables and add to the broth.
3. Cook 5 to 10 minutes and serve.
* You may substitute canned beans and lentils provided you rinse and drain beans well.

TOOSHI'S DINNER

INGREDIENTS:
Select 6 oz., in total, of one or more of the following meats-

Shrimp	Turkey cutlet	Chicken liver
Scallops	Chicken cutlet	

3 tomatoes
One fresh garlic
One onion
6 mushrooms
1/4 cup bean sprouts
Spices you like
½ cup red wine or 1 cup water with ½ tablespoon corn oil

DIRECTIONS:

1. Heat a frying pan for one minute. Add ½ cup wine or 1 cup water with ½ tablespoon corn oil along with your choice of meat (cutlets should be chopped into bite sized pieces).

2. Cover and cook on medium high heat for 8 to 10 minutes.

3. Drain off water if water was added. Add spices, mix well. Continue to cook with lid off until meat becomes lightly browned.

4. Chop all vegetables, add to the meat.

5. Cover and cook over medium heat 6 to 8 minutes and serve.

TOOSHI'S PILAF

INGREDIENTS:
One cup dry rice
½ cup snow peas or green beans
One large bell pepper
½ chopped red onion

½ cup chopped parsley
One tablespoon corn oil
One and one-half cups water
DIRECTIONS:
1. In a sauce pan, bring the water to a boil.
2. Add cup of rice, stir well. Lower heat and cook 20 minutes or until firm.
3. Place all vegetables into a second sauce pan, add some water. Cook 5 minutes.
4. Drain water.
5. Serve vegetables over the rice.

TOOSHI'S SAUCE

INGREDIENTS:
2 tomatoes
One fresh garlic
5 mushrooms
One teaspoon corn oil
One tablespoon grated cheese
Spices you like (oregano, basil)
DIRECTIONS:
1. Heat a frying pan for one minute.
2. Add chopped tomatoes and corn oil. Cover and cook 5 minutes over medium heat or until all the juice comes out of the tomatoes.
3. Add grated cheese. Stir well.
4. Add chopped mushroom and garlic. Mix well. Cover and cook another 5 minutes over low heat and serve over meat, rice or spaghetti.

TOOSHI'S SHISH-KA-BAB

INGREDIENTS:
6 oz chicken cutlet
2 tomatoes
6 mushrooms
One onion
1/4 cup wine
Spices you like
DIRECTIONS:
1. Cut cutlet into cubes.
2. Cut vegetables into wedges.
3. Arrange cutlet, tomato, mushroom and onion alternately on a spear.
4. Add spices and marinate in wine.
5. Bake in oven or over grill until meat is roasted.

TOOSHI'S SOUP

INGREDIENTS:
Select either chicken or turkey cutlet or chicken liver (total 4 oz)
Celery, carrots, cabbage, tomato, onion, scallion. Swiss chard
Spinach, mushroom, parsley, dill, kale
Barley and lentils (1/4 cup for each person)
One fresh lemon
Spices you like
DIRECTIONS:
1. Chop the meat into small pieces.
2. Add to a deep soup pot along with barley and lentils and two cups of water.
3. Cook for 10 minutes after bringing to a boil.
4. Add chopped vegetables, lemon wedges and corn oil.
5. Cook another 15 minutes with lid on over medium heat and serve.

TOOSHI'S STEW

INGREDIENTS:
1/4 pound 90% lean ground beef or chicken cutlet
½ zucchini
½ eggplant
One medium onion
One tomato
One green pepper
One cup string beans
One whole garlic
One cup water
Spices you like (hot pepper, oregano)
DIRECTIONS:
1. Bring one cup water to a boil in a deep pot.
2. Add beef or *cutlet (cubed). Cook 10 minutes on medium heat.
3. Chop and add all vegetables. Cook another 10 minutes with lid on.
4. Stir well and serve.
* If selecting chicken cutlet, add one tablespoon corn oil in Step 2.

VEGETARIAN DINNER

INGREDIENTS:
½ zucchini
2 tomatoes
One cup each chopped spinach, broccoli, string beans, mushrooms
One whole garlic
Two slices low fat cheese (Alpine Lace cheese)
½ cup water
Spices you like

DIRECTIONS:
1. Cut all vegetables. Add to deep frying pan or soup pot. Add water and corn oil.
2. Cover and cook 8 minutes over medium to high heat.
3. Reduce heat, mix well, drain excess water.
4. Add seasonings and simmer another 5 minutes.
5. Place vegetables on dinner plate. Add two slices cheese as a topping.
6. After cheese has melted. Serve.

VEGETARIAN II

INGREDIENTS:
A variety of beans (*dry or canned)
Tooshi's Sauce
One tomato
6 mushrooms
3 oz cheese
One onion
Seasonings you like
DIRECTIONS:
1. Soak or rinse beans (*soak dry beans 5—6 hours before cooking).
2. Cook in 2 cups water for 5 minutes.
3. Drain off water. Set aside.
4. Prepare Tooshi's Sauce, add 3 oz low fat cheese to the sauce.
5. Add the Tooshi's Sauce to the beans. Cover and simmer 5 minutes and serve.

VEGGIE SHRIMP

INGREDIENTS:
5—7 large shrimp
1/3 cup broccoli
½ cup carrots
5 mushrooms
½ cup spinach
One tomato
One tablespoon corn oil
Spices you like
DIRECTIONS:
1. Place shrimp onto aluminum foil.
2. Add corn oil and vegetables.
3. Fold foil and cook in oven at 350 for 20—25 minutes and serve.

YUPPIE'S DELIGHT

INGREDIENTS:
4 oz flounder
3 shrimp
1 lemon
Tooshi's Sauce (3-4 tablespoons)
Spices—basil and pepper
DIRECTIONS:
1. Place the fish and shrimp onto aluminum foil.
2. Add spices and sliced lemon over seafood.
3. Add Tooshi's Sauce. Wrap foil tightly.
4. Bake at 350 for 20—25 minutes and serve.

CHAPTER 15

HIGH CALORIE SNACK FOODS

Snack foods from vending machines are divided into 3 groups.
  A) *Snacks over 250 calories:*
    Snickers Bar
    Butterfinger
    Baby Ruth
    Three Musketeers
    Mr. Goodbar
  B) *Snacks between 200—250 calories:*
    M&M Plain
    Reese's Peanut Butter Cups
    Pay Day
    Hershey Bar with Almonds
    Almond Joy
    Nestle Crunch
    Kit Kat
    Milky Way (dark)
    Planter's Cheese/Peanut Butter Sandwiches
    M&M's Peanuts

C) *Snacks under 200 calories:*
   Cheetos Cheese Puffs
   Twix
   Snack-Ems Snack Mix
   Famous Amos Chocolate Chip Cookies
   Act II Microwave Popcorn
   Frito's Corn Chips
   Oreo Cookies
   Lay's Potato Chips
   Dorito's Nacho Cheese Tortilla Chips
    Nature Valley Oats-N-Honey Granola Bar
   Cheeze-it

CONSTITUENTS OF 100 GRAMS
OF VARIOUS FOODS

NAME	CAL-ORIES	PROTEIN	FAT	CARBO-HYDRATES	SODIUM
DAIRY PRODUCTS:					
Cheese					
Blue mold	368	21.5	30.5	2.0	—-
Cheddar	398	2.0	32.2	2.1	700
Cheddar (processed)	370	23.2	29.9	2.2	1500
Cottage	95	19.5	5	2.0	290
Cream Cheese	371	9.0	37.0	2.0	250
Swiss	370	27.5	28.0	1.7	710

Swiss (processed)	355	26.4	26.9	1.6	—-

Milk (cow)

Fluid —Whole	68	3.5	3.9	4.9	50
Fluid —Non-fat	36	3.5	.1	5.1	52

FATS, OILS, SHORTENINGS:

Butter	716	.6	81	.4	980
Margarine	720	.6	81	.4	1100
Mayonnaise	708	1.5	78	3.0	590
Oils (salad / cooking)	884	0	100	0	.2
Salad Dressing (French)	394	.6	35.5	20.3	——

FRUITS:

Blackberries (raw)	57	1.2	1.0	12.5	.2
Blueberries (raw)	61	.6	.6	15.1	.6
Blueberries (cnd.,sweet)	98	.4	.4	26	——
Cranberry sauce (cnd.)	198	.1	.3	51.4	1

Name	Calories	Protein	Fat	Carbohydrates	Sodium
Raspberries, red (frozen)	98	.7	.2	24.7	.7
Strawberries (raw)	37	.8	.5	8.3	.8
Grapefruit (raw)	40	.5	.2	10.1	.5
Grapefruit (cnd.,sweet)	72	.6	.2	19.1	——
Lemons	32	.9	.6	8.7	.7
Limes	37	.8	.1	12.3	1
Oranges	45	.9	.2	11.2	.3
Tangerines	44	.8	.3	10.9	2
Cantaloupes	20	.6	.2	4.6	12
Honey Dew	32	.5	0	8.5	—
Watermelon	28	.5	.2	6.9	.3

NAME	CAL-ORIES	PROTEIN	FAT	CARBO-HYDRATES	SODIUM
Fruits (cont.):					
Apples (raw)	58	.3	.4	14.9	.2
Apples (dry,unckd.)	277	1.4	1.0	73.2	—
Apricots (raw)	51	1.0	.1	12.9	.6

Apricots (cnd.,swt.)	80	.6	.1	21.4	2
Apricots (dry)	262	5.2	.4	66.9	11
Avocado	245	1.7	26.4	5.1	3
Bananas	88	1.2	.2	23	.5
Cherries	61	1.1	.5	14.8	1
Cherries (cnd.)	48	.8	.3	11.9	3
Dates (dried)	284	2.2	.6	75.4	1
Figs (cnd.,swt.)	113	.8	.3	30.0	1
Figs (dried)	270	4.0	1.2	68.4	34
Papaya (raw)	43	.6	.1	10.0	—
Peaches (raw)	46	.5	.1	12.0	.5
Pears (raw)	63	.7	.4	15.8	2
Pears (cnd.,swt.)	68	.2	.1	18.4	8
Plums (raw)	50	.7	.2	12.2	.6
Prunes (dry)	268	2.3	.6	71.0	6
Raisins	268	2.3	.5	71.2	21

FRUIT JUICES AND OTHER FRUIT PRODUCTS:

Apple Juice	50	.1	0	13.8	4
Apple Sauce	72	.2	.1	19.7	.3
Grape Juice	67	.4	0	18.2	1
Olives, green (jar)	132	1.5	13.5	4.0	2400
Olives, ripe	191	1.8	21.0	2.6	980
Orange Juice (fresh)	44	.8	.2	11.0	3.6
Orange Juice (cnd.)	44	.8	.2	11.1	400
Pineapple Juice	49	.3	.1	13.9	.4
Pineapple Juice (cnd.)	49	.3	.1	13.9	400
Prune Juice (cnd.)	71	.4	0	19.3	450
Tomato Juice (cnd.)	21	1.0	.2	4.3	250

GRAINS AND GRAIN PRODUCTS:

Breakfast Cereals

Bran Flakes	292	10.8	1.9	78.8	1400
Corn Flakes	385	8.1	.4	85.0	660
Farina	44	1.3	.1	9.1	11

| Oatmeal | 63 | 2.3 | 1.2 | 11.0 | .3 |
| Oat Breakfast Cereal | 396 | 14.5 | 7.0 | 70.2 | —— |

NAME	CAL- ORIES	PROTEIN	FAT	CARBO- HYDRATES	SODIUM
Breakfast Cereal (cont.)					
Puffed Rice	392	5.9	.6	87.7	.9
Puffed Wheat	355	10.8	1.6	80.2	4
Rice Flakes	392	5.9	.6	87.7	720
Wheat Flakes	355	10.8	1.6	80.2	1300

FLOURS, MEALS AND OTHER FARINACEOUS MATERIALS:

Wheat	350	9.2	1.0	73.8	1500
Flour, all purpose	364	10.5	1.0	76.1	1
Rice, brown	360	7.5	1.7	77.7	9
Rice, converted	362	7.6	.3	79.4	4
Rice, white	362	7.6	.3	79.4	2
Starch, pure	362	.5	.2	87	4
Tapioca, dry	360	.6	.2	86.4	5

Wild Rice	364	14.1	.7	75.3	7
Wheat Germ	361	25.2	10.0	49.5	2
Spaghetti, cooked	149	5.1	.6	30.2	—

BAKED AND COOKED PRODUCTS:

Breads

Cracked Wheat	259	8.5	2.2	51.4	620
French or Vienna	270	8.1	2.7	52.0	—
Raisin	284	7.1	3.1	57.8	—
Rye	244	9.1	1.2	52.4	590
White	275	8.5	3.2	51.8	640
Whole Wheat	240	9.3	2.6	49.0	930
Rolls, plain	309	9.0	5.5	55.1	—

Cakes and Pies

Angel Food	270	8.4	.3	58.7	—
Foundation	350	5.9	11.7	55.9	—
Fruit Cake	354	5.2	11.7	55.9	—
Plain	327	6.4	8.2	57.0	—
Corn Bread	219	6.7	4.7	36.6	—

Name	Calories	Protein	Fat	Carbohydrates	Sodium
Crackers, Graham	393	8.0	10.0	74.3	710
Crackers, Saltines	431	9.2	11.8	71.1	1100
Donuts	425	6.6	21.0	52.7	—
Fig Bars	350	4.2	4.8	75.8	—
Apple	246	2.1	9.5	39.5	—
Pumpkin	202	4.6	9.6	25.8	—
Pretzels	369	8.8	3.2	74.5	1700

NAME	CAL-ORIES	PROTEIN	FAT	CARBO-HYDRATES	SODIUM
NUTS AND NUT PRODUCTS:					
Almonds	597	18.6	54.1	19.6	160
Brazil Nuts	646	14.4	65.9	11.0	1
Cashews, roasted	578	18.5	48.2	27.0	200
Peanuts, roasted	559	26.9	44.2	23.6	460
Peanut Butter	576	26.1	47.8	21.0	120
Pecans	696	9.4	73.0	13.0	.3
Walnuts	654	15.0	64.4	15.6	2

MEAT, POULTRY AND SEAFOOD:

Beef Chuck, cooked	309	26	22	0	51
Hamburger, cooked	364	22	30	0	107
Round, cooked	233	27	13	0	68
Corned Beef (cnd.)	216	25.3	12	0	1300
Roast Beef	224	25	13	0	——
Lamb, Leg, roast	235	18.0	17.5	0	78
Pork, bacon, fried	607	25	55	1	2400
Pork, Canadian	231	22.1	15	.3	—
Ham, fresh	344	15.2	31	0	—
Ham, cured	397	23	33	.4	1100
Pork, luncheon	289	14.9	24.3	1.5	—
Veal Cutlet	219	28	11	0	—
Liver, beef	136	19.7	3.2	6.0	110
Bluefish, baked	155	27.4	4.2	0	—
Caviar, Sturgeon	243	26.9	15.0—		—

Clams	81	12.8	1.4	3.4	180
Cod	74	16.5	.4	0	60
Crabs, canned	104	16.9	2.9	1.3	1000
Flounder	68	14.9	.5	0	—
Halibut	126	18.6	5.2	0	56
Herring	191	18.3	12.5	0	——
Lobster	88	16.2	1.9	.5	210
Oysters	84	9.8	2.1	5.6	73
Salmon, raw	223	17.4	16.5	0	48
Salmon, canned	203	19.7	3.2	0	540
Sardines, canned	214	25.7	11.0	1.2	510
Scallops Shrimp, raw	78	14.8	.1	3.4	150
Shrimp, canned	127	26.8	1.4	—	140
Swordfish	178	27.4	6.8	0	—
Tuna fish, canned	198	29.0	8.2	0	800

NAME	CAL-ORIES	PROTEIN	FAT	CARBO-HYDRATES	SODIUM
EGGS AND POULTRY:					
Chicken, roaster	200	20.2	12.6	0	110
Chicken Liver	141	22.1	4.0	2.6	51
Turkey	268	20.1	20.2	0	40-92
Eggs, Whole	162	12.8	11.5	.7	81
SUGARS AND SWEETS:					
Chocolate milk	503	6.0	33.5	55.7	86
Hard candy	383	0	0	99.0	—
Cocoa, breakfast	293	8	23.8	48.9	57
Jams & Marmalades	278	.5	.3	70.8	7-13
Sugar, cane or beet	385	0	0	99.5	.3
Sugar, brown	370	0	0	95.5	24

VEGETABLES:

Carrots, raw	42	1.2	.3	9.3	51
Potatoes, white, baked	83	2.0	.1	19.1	.8
Radishes	20	1.2	.1	4.2	9
Turnips	32	1.1	.2	7.1	58
Asparagus, raw	21	2.2	.2	3.9	2
Asparagus, canned	18	1.9	.3	2.9	410
Beet greens	27	2.0	.3	5.6	130
Brussel sprouts	47	4.4	.5	8.9	11
Cabbage	24	1.4	.2	5.3	5
Sauerkraut	22	1.4	.3	4.4	630
Swiss Chard	27	2.6	.4	4.8	84
Chicory	21	1.6	.3	2.9	—
Chives	52	3.8	.6	7.8	—
Kale	40	3.9	.6	7.2	110
Lettuce	15	1.2	.2	2.9	12
Mustard Greens	22	2.3	.3	4.0	48
Onions	45	1.4	.2	10.3	1
Spinach, raw	20	2.3	.3	3.2	82

Red Kidney Beans	336	23.1	1.7	59.4	—
Lima Beans	128	7.5	.8	23.5	680
Broccoli	29	3.3	.2	5.5	400
Chick Peas	359	20.8	4.7	60.9	—
Corn, cob	92	3.7	1.2	20.5	.4
Cucumber	12	.7	.1	2.7	.9
Eggplant	24	1.1	.2	5.5	.9
Lentils, dry	339	24.0	1.2	60.4	3
Mushrooms, raw	16	2.4	.3	4.0	5

NAME	CAL- ORIES	PROTEIN	FAT	CARBO- HYDRATES	SODIUM
Vegetables (cont.)					
Peas, green, raw	98	6.7	.4	17.7	1
Peas, green, frozen	83	5.7	.4	12.9	160
Pumpkin, raw	31	1.2	.2	7.3	.6
Soy Beans, dry	331	34.9	18.1	34.8	4

Squash, winter, raw	38	1.5	.3	8.8	.3
Squash, summer, raw	16	.6	.1	3.9	.2
Tomatoes, raw	20	1.0	.3	4.0	3
Tomato ketchup	98	2.0	.4	24.5	1300

CALORIC EXPENDITURE
OF
PHYSICAL ACTIVITIES

Aerobics (medium)	340
Badminton	350
Basketball (vigorous)	680
Bicycling (5.5 MPH)	203
Bowling	202
Calisthenics (light)	272
Cleaning	253
Cycling (13 MPH)	680
Disco Dancing	307
Fencing	292
Football (touch)	470
Gardening	215
Gardening (raking)	218
Golf	244
Horseback riding (trotting)	348
Housework (cleaning)	271
Ice skating (10 MPH)	394

Jogging (medium)	610
Lawn Mowing (hand)	267
Lawn Moving (power)	244
Racquetball (social)	544
Roller skating	347
Running or jogging (10 MPH)	944
Skiing (10 MPH)	597
Square Dancing	346
Swimming (.25 MPH)	298
Table Tennis	350
Tennis	410
Volleyball	344
Walking (2.5 MPH)	204
Walking (3.75 MPH)	300
Weight Lifting (heavy)	612
Wood chopping/sawing	394

MEASUREMENTS

LENGTH

12 Inches	=1 foot
3 feet	=1 yard
1,760 yards	=1 mile

AREA

10,000 sq. miles	=2.47 acres
1 acre	=4,000 sq. meters
1 sq. mile	=2.6 sq. kilometers

METRIC SYSTEM

10 millimeters	=	1 centimeter
100 centimeters	=	1 meter
1000 meters	=	1 kilometer
1 inch	=	2.54 centimeters
1 foot	=	0.305 meter

1 yard	=	0.915 meter
1 mile	=	1,609 meters

WEIGHT

16 ounces	=	1 pound
112 pounds	=	1 CWT.
20 CWT.	=	1 Ton

LIQUID MEASURE

4 gills	=	1 Pint
2 pints	=	1 quart
4 quarts	=	1 gallon
1 liter	=	13/4 pints
1 pint	=	0.568 liter
1 gallon	=	4.55 liters

TEMPERATURE

BOILING POINT

Celsius	100
Fahrenheit	212

FREEZING

Celsius	0
Fahrenheit	32

CONVERSION

Celsius X 9/5+32   =Fahrenheit
Fahrenheit X 5/9-32   =Celsius

About the Book

Of all the factors that influence our life and upon which our health and illness depend, undoubtedly the nature of the food we eat is the most important. That is why we find in our contemporary society men, women and even children struggling to control their weight.

With Dr. Tooshi's Diet you will lose weight quickly and safely. More importantly, Dr. Tooshi has helped thousands of people to lose weight successfully. He has included his personal techniques and instructions so that you, too, may benefit from his 20 years of practical experience in the field of weight loss. Included in his book is a basic course in Public Health Nutrition, a comprehensive exercise program and his personal collection of weight loss recipes. Dr. Tooshi's weight loss program is truly the first comprehensive approach to losing weight and keeping it off for many years to come.

About the Author

Dr. Alan M. Tooshi received his Masters of Science degree from Southern Illinois University and his Ph.D. from the University of Illinois. Upon his graduation in 1970, he took a teaching position at the New Jersey City University. Since then he has been teaching Public Health Nutrition, Epidemiology, Mental Health and Weight Management to both graduate and undergraduate students. Dr. Tooshi has written his doctoral thesis "The Effects of Exercise on the Blood Cholesterol, Blood Pressure and Body Composition."

In 1980, Dr. Tooshi organized the Hudson Diet Clinic in Bayonne, New Jersey, where he has been planning diets for people who want to lose weight as well as for people who have medical problems such as heart disease, diabetes and digestive disorders. He currently practices in Howell, New Jersey. Dr. Tooshi speaks and lectures on nutrition, weight loss, exercise, and stress reduction.